A Brief History of Opium

Mythology, Culture, Medicine, Trade, and Conflict

Matthew Leigh Embleton

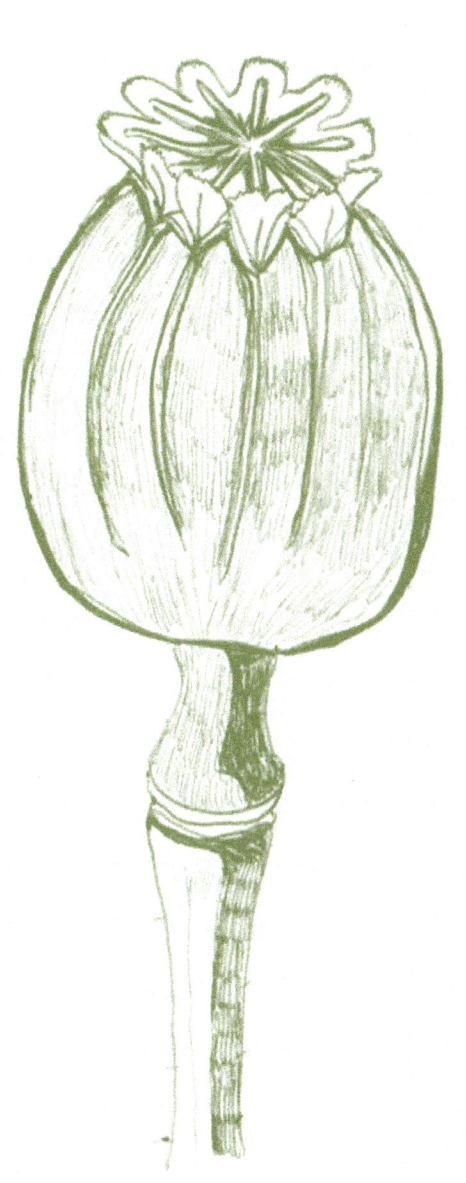

Copyright ©2021 Matthew Leigh Embleton. All rights reserved.

A Brief History of Opium

1. Ancient Times: *The Search for Origins (before 800 BCE)* 1
2. Antiquity: *Dark Mythology and the Light of Science (800 BCE-476 CE)* 8
   2.1 Dark Mythology 8
   2.2 The Light of Science 15
3. The Middle Ages: *East-West Exchange (476-1453)* 20
4. Early Modern Times: *Renaissance (1453-1800)* 24
   4.1 The Near East: The Ottoman World 24
   4.2 The Far East: Chinese Dominance 26
   4.3 Europe: Alchemy and Science 27
   4.4 New Trade Routes to the East 32
   4.5 Opium and Romanticism, Part 1 35
5. The 19th Century Part 1: *Culture, Science, and Art (1800-1839)* 38
   5.1 Opium in the East: The Smoking Ritual 38
   5.2 Opium in the West: Science and Addiction 40
   5.3 Opium and Romanticism, Part 2 42
6. The Opium Wars: *East and West Collide (1839-1860)* 44
   6.1 Diplomacy and Trade 44
   6.2 The Crackdown on Opium 48
   6.3 Voices of Opposition 50
   6.4 The First Opium War 51
   6.5 The Second Opium War 52
7. The 19th Century Part 2: *Danger, Addiction, and Vice (1850-1900)* 56
   7.1 Science and 'God's Own Medicine' 56
   7.2 From East to West: The Spread of Opium Culture 59
   7.3 Opium and Romanticism, Part 3 63
8. Modern Times: *Drugs, War, and Politics (1900-Present)* 64
   8.1 Medicine and Addiction 64
   8.2 Regulation and Prohibition in the United States 65
   8.3 Regulation and Prohibition in Britain 67
   8.4 Regulation and Prohibition in China 67
   8.5 Organised Crime in the United States: The Commission 67
   8.6 Organised Crime in Europe: The Corsican Mafia 68
   8.7 Organised Crime in China: The Green Gang 69
   8.8 Southeast Asia and the Golden Triangle 70
   8.9 The French Connection 70
   8.10 CAT and Air America 75
   8.11 The War on Drugs 76
   8.12 The Golden Crescent 76
   8.13 Today 78
   8.14 Popular Culture 80

Cover: Papaver Somniferum, Illustration by the Author

All images in this book are sourced from Wikipedia Creative Commons and are in the public domain, unless otherwise specified.

Acknowledgments

I have long been fascinated by languages and history, and I am very grateful to the special people in my life who have supported and encouraged me in my work. Thank you for believing in me. You know who you are.

Thanks to Historian, Assyriologist, and Egyptologist Dr Andrea Sinclair for her correspondence and feedback regarding the 'Ancient Times' chapter of this book.

Introduction

The origin of humankind's relationship with the opium poppy is complex, and the further back in time we look, the more speculation we find filling in the gaps. This strange and mysterious plant has the power to inspire the imagination, as much in the study of its history, as when the Romantic Poets used its extracts to stimulate their imagination to write their poetry.

From ancient civilisations to the present day, the opium poppy (Papaver Somniferum) has a fascinating history, from the dark symbolism of trance, sleep, dreams, and death in Greco-Roman mythology, to the search for ever stronger pain relief. Since its discovery as a powerful painkiller in ancient medical texts, to the battlefields of the American Civil War, 'God's Own Medicine' has been both a blessing and a curse.

The growth of the opium trade has caused and funded wars. It has both relieved pain, and been the cause of pain and suffering. Its illicit use, addiction, and surrounding war and politics have plagued humankind to this day.

There is no more effective painkiller than that which has its origins in this beautiful plant. There is also little in the way of medicine which carries with it such dangers of addiction, ruin, misery and death. Attempts by scientists to isolate and refine opium to safely regulate its dosage and reduce addiction, have unwittingly opened a Pandora's box of consequences which have gone on to shape the modern world.

In ancient mythology, this opium giving plant could be seen as a gift from the gods. But like those cautionary tales revealing the flaws in human nature, such a gift comes at a great price.

This book is a brief introduction to the history of opium from its earliest beginnings to modern times. Its chapters break this history down into periods of historical significance. Each chapter carries its own different themes and episodes in the overall story of civilisation, humankind, and its relationship with nature.

1. Ancient Times: *The Search for Origins (before 800 BCE)*

It has long been thought that the beginnings of the poppy can be found in the so called 'Fertile Crescent', one of the cradles of civilisation which emerged from 9000-7500 BCE, from around the eastern Mediterranean Basin, stretching some 1,800 miles from Ancient Egypt, up along the Levant to Phoenicia, Assyria, along the southern border of the Anatolian and Armenian highlands, and down the Tigris and Euphrates of Mesopotamia to the Persian Gulf. This is one of the places where people first began to clear spaces of land of their natural vegetation to grow crops, developing systems of irrigation and other technological innovations that caused civilisation to flourish.

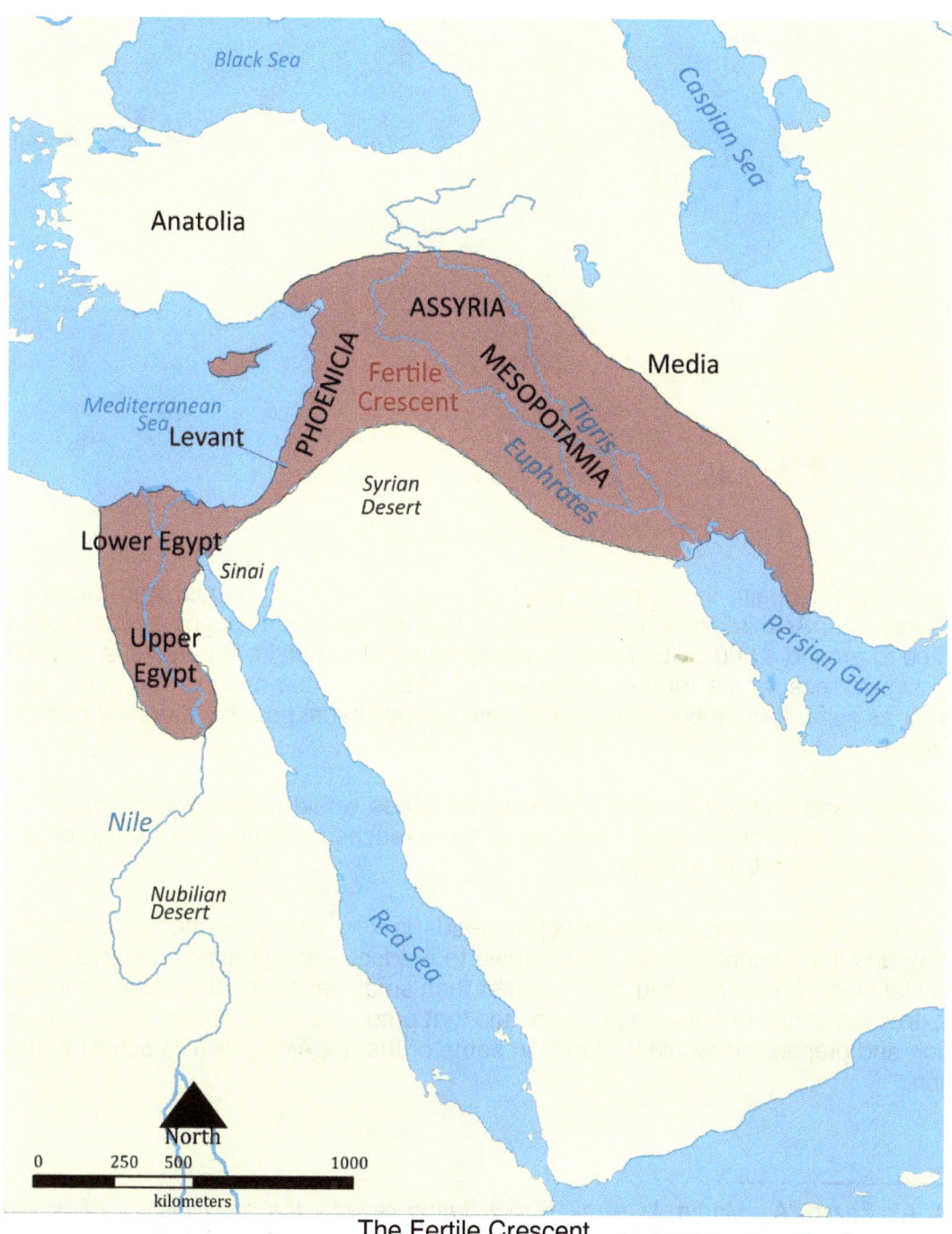

The Fertile Crescent

The development of agriculture spread across the Mediterranean and Europe, and scientific studies indicate that the opium poppy (*Papaver Somniferum*) was being cultivated by around 5500 BCE in the central and western Mediterranean, spreading to north western temperate Europe and the western Alps by 5000-4500 BCE.[1]

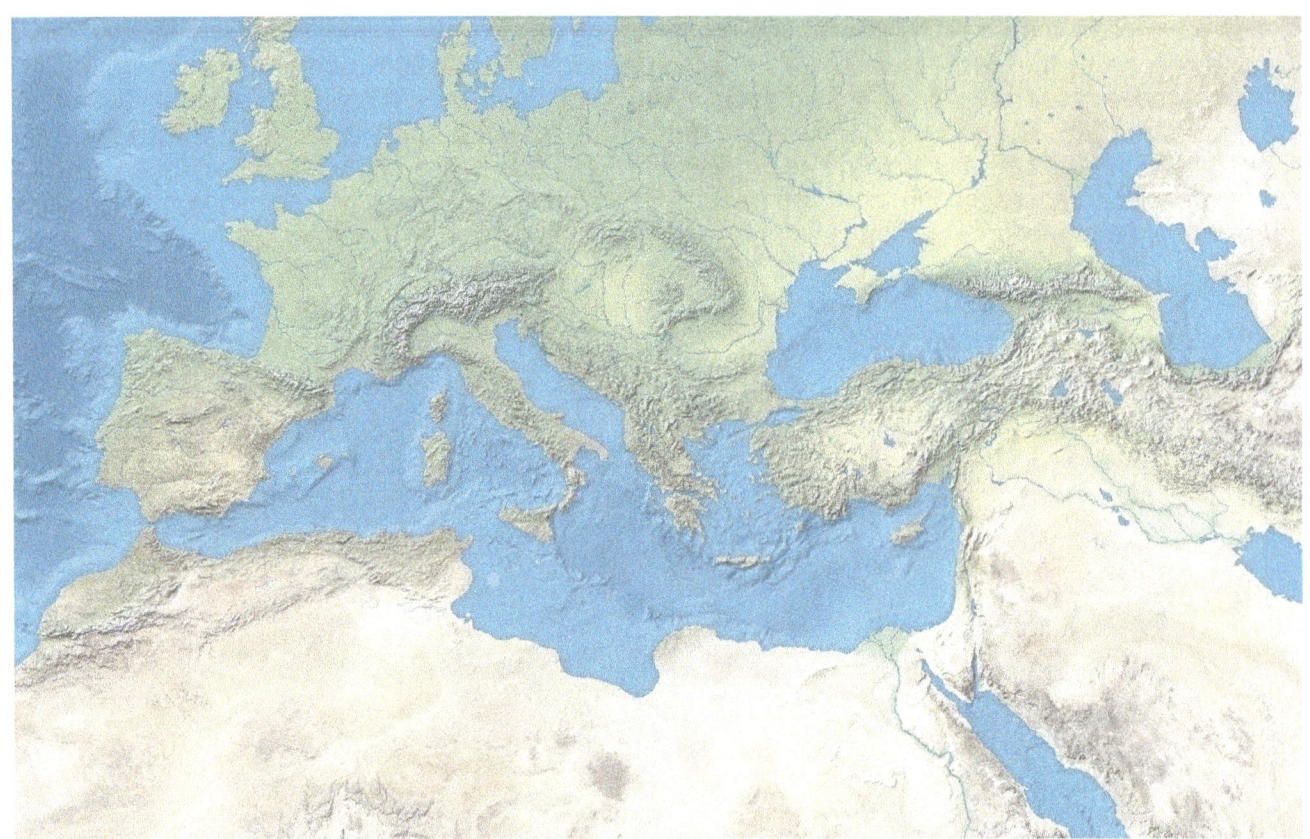

The Mediterranean and the Near East

In Zuheros, southern Spain, the 'Cave of Bats' (*Cueva de los Murciélagos*) was found to contain a Neolithic burial site. At this site small deposits of toasted grain and poppy seeds were found and carbon dated to around 4,200 BCE. These deposits found at a burial site suggest a possible religious or spiritual significance, in the form of some kind of offering to the dead or the gods, either in their plain form, or as some form of bread decorated with poppy seeds, possibly eaten as part of some sort of sacred meal.

Some have theorised that the toasting of the poppy seeds would have given off opium fumes, with which some kind of shaman or oracle figure would have reached a trance-like state in order to be able to communicate with the dead or divine.

The amount of opium alkaloids found in poppy seeds is very little (it is measured in billionths of a gram, 10^{-9}g), and the amount it would take to toast to produce enough fumes capable of inducing any trance-like state would have resulted in tons rather than small deposits being found at the site. If there was any extraction of opium from the poppy heads that produced those seeds, then perhaps traces of its collection and preparation would be found in some of the '*La Almagra*' (red ochre) pottery found in that location.

---

[1] Salavert, A., Zazzo, A., Martin, L. et al. *Direct dating reveals the early history of opium poppy in western Europe.* Sci Rep 10, 20263 (2020). https://doi.org/10.1038/s41598-020-76924-3

The Sumerians in lower Mesopotamia are often credited as being the first people to have domesticated the poppy in around c3400 BCE. The theory is based on a claim that the Sumerian texts referred to the opium poppy as 'Hul Gil' (the 'joy plant'). This would have been at a time when cuneiform was still in the early stages of development away from pictographic proto-writing. However, the specialist fields of Egyptology and Assyriology can find no conclusive textual or visual evidence to support this theory.

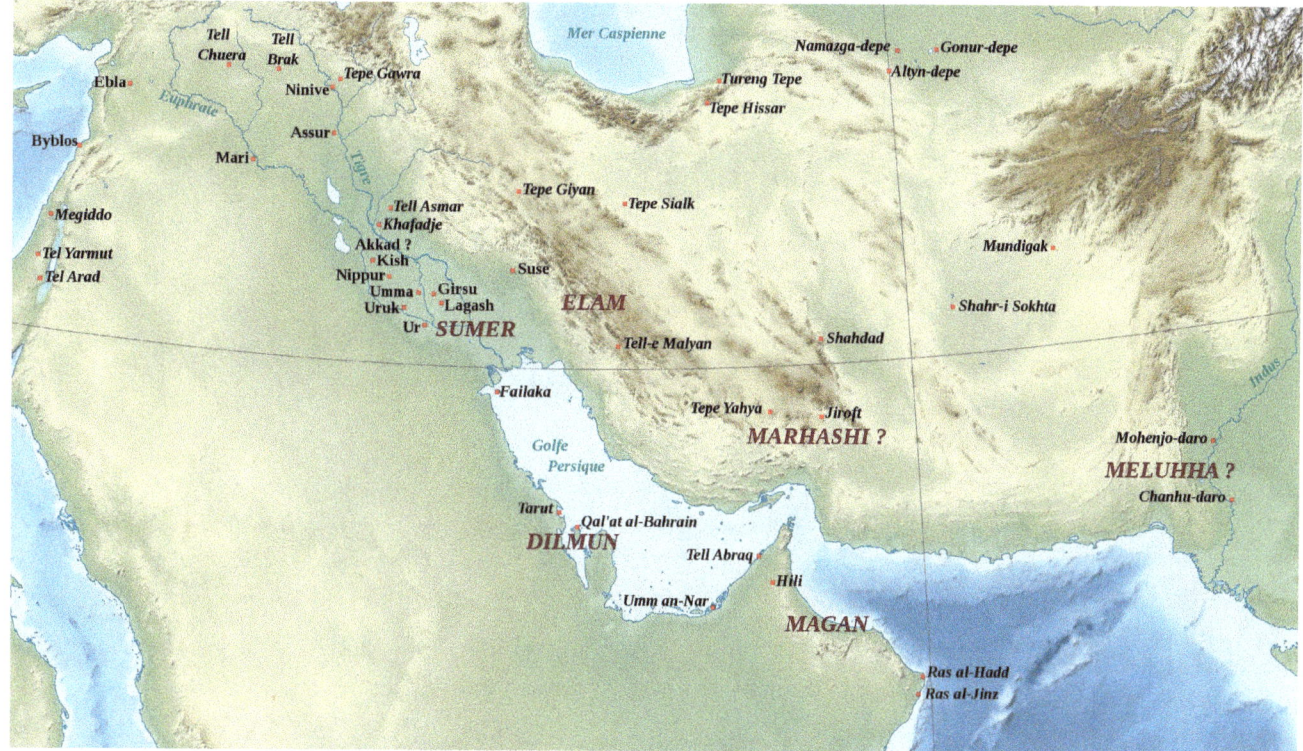

The Middle East, 3rd Millennium BCE

The Assyriologist A. P. Dougherty, a professor at Yale University is credited with the translation, but cautioned that "Gil as a single ideogram represented a number of plants", and "its meaning in the ideogram for 'opium' is difficult to determine with exactness". This caution was not heeded, and the translation has been used, re-used, and cited in many books and articles. At best, the combination 'Hul Gil' is more likely to mean a 'stink' or a 'bitter cucumber'.

Another claim is that the Nippur Tablet, which has been dated to around c2100-2000 BCE, contains text which describes the practice of collecting poppy juice in the morning and its use in the production of opium. However, the translation of the tablet that this idea was based on has since been rejected. At best, the symbols used are more likely to mean a type of marsh or reed rush.[2]

Nippur was an important spiritual centre for the Sumerians. It had temples dedicated to many deities, including the shrine of Enlil, the chief deity of the Sumerian pantheon who was also the god of wind, air, earth, and storms. Perhaps because of the sacred city status of Nippur at this time, and the religious and spiritual activity that must have taken place there, it has lent itself to the idea in some minds that anywhere where there are rituals in the ancient world, there must have been some kind of mind-altering substance used as part of that ritual, and therefore, if it was happening anywhere, it must have been happing in Nippur.

---

[2] Sinclair, A. [Updated April 2021]. *Hul Gil and the opium poppy: A comedy of errors* [online]. Available from: http://artisticlicenseorwhyitrustnoone.blogspot.com/2020/12/hul-gil-and-opium-poppy-comedy-of-errors.html [Accessed July 2021

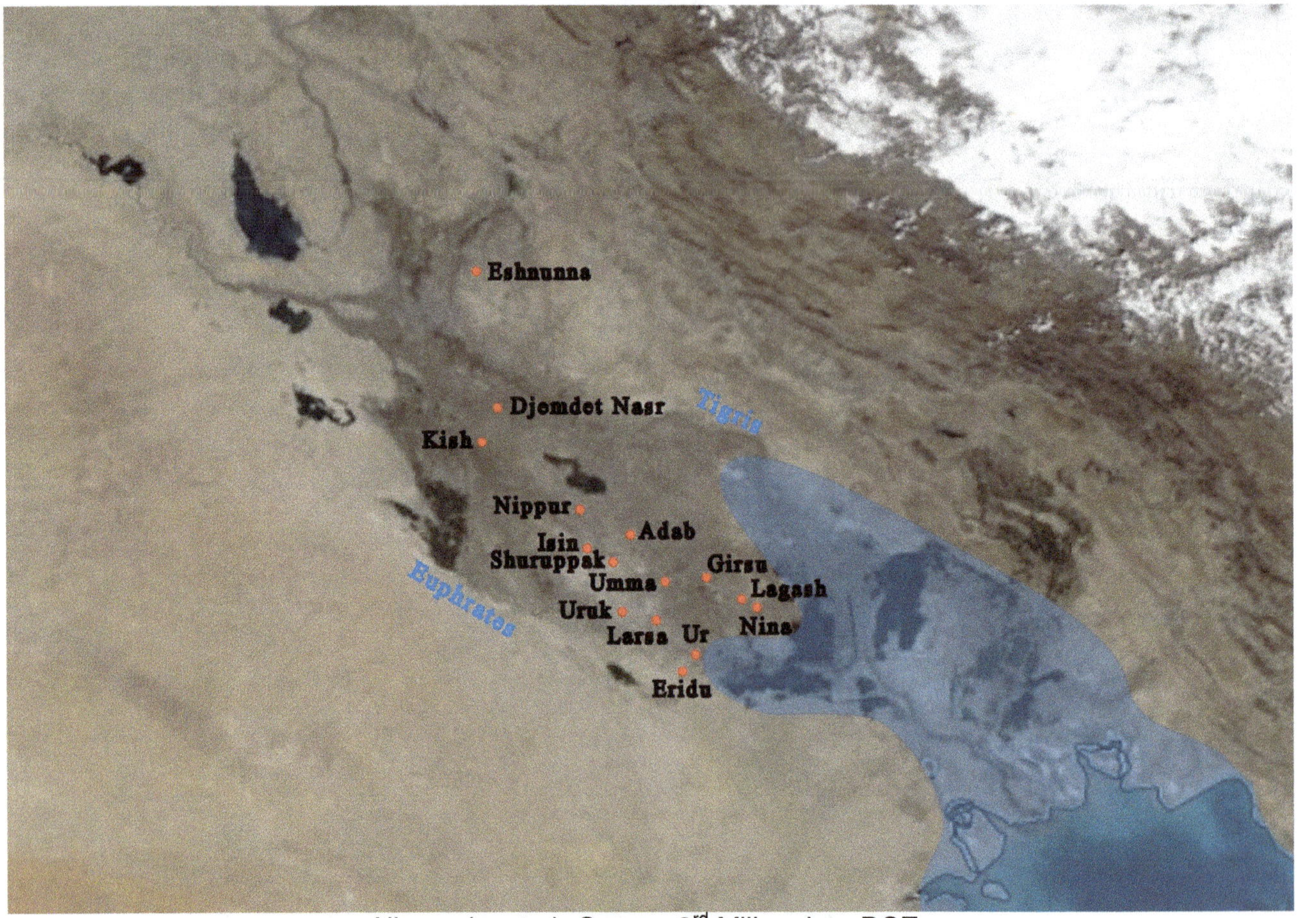

Nippur (centre), Sumer, 3rd Millennium BCE

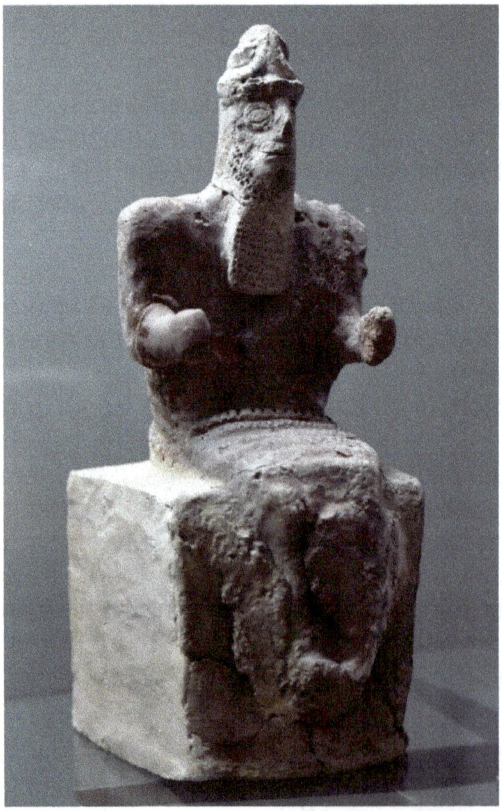

The ancient Mesopotamian god 'Enlil', c1800-1600 BCE

The Ebers Papyrus is one of the most important medical documents in the history of ancient Egyptian medicine. It is dated to around 1550 BCE and contains herbal remedies collected from other older texts, with over 800 magical formulas, remedies, and healing charms.

While this document has often been referenced as proof of the use of opium in ancient Egyptian medicine, only a handful of the remedies are thought to refer to the poppy as an ingredient, these are based on translations which are disputed by some scholars, and they may only refer to the use of the poppy seeds.[3]

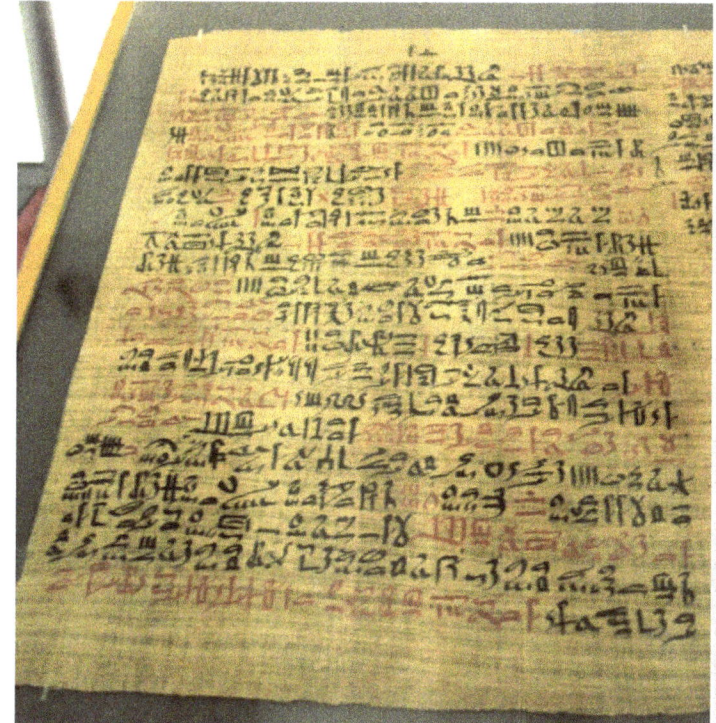
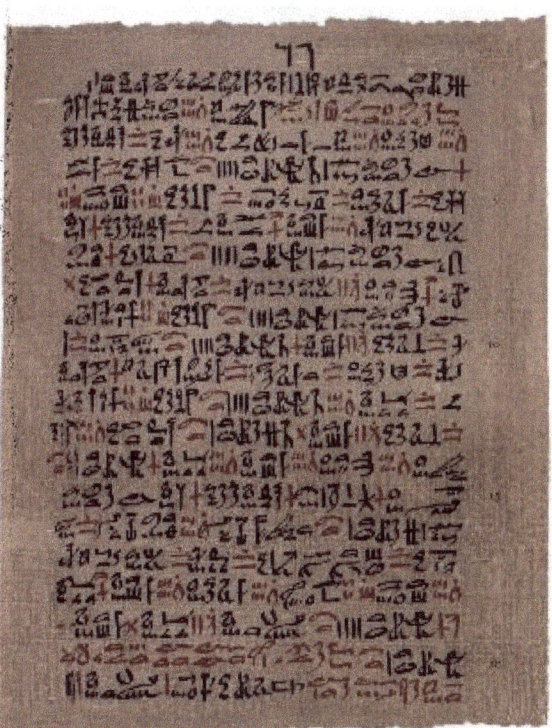

The Ebers Papyrus

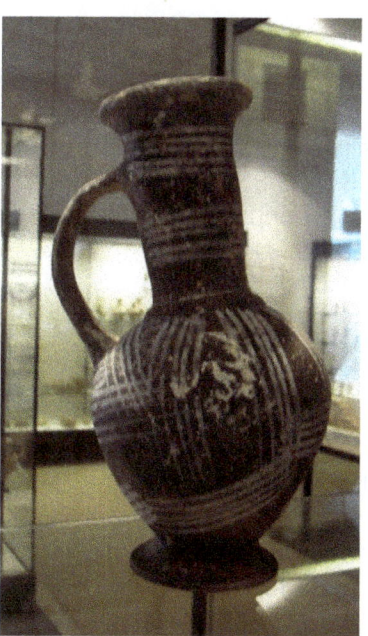

During the Late Bronze Age (c1650-1350 BCE) Cyprus produced and exported large amounts of pottery, influenced by the latest Mycenaean designs. Some of these jugs known as 'base-ring juglets' were fashioned in the shape of poppy heads. This has led to suggestions that some of them contained opium.

Scientific analysis of residues found in excavated pottery from this period, found that small traces of opium alkaloids were detected in plant oils.

This led some to conclude that along with a wide trade in pottery, there was also a well-established trade in opium by this time, and that opium was used in religious rituals dating to approximately 1000 BCE.

Poppy seeds themselves contain small traces of opium alkaloids, and the plant oils could have been part of a mixture, of which poppy seed oil was present. This could have been used for religious purposes such as anointing, or as perfume.

---

[3] Sinclair, A. [2021].

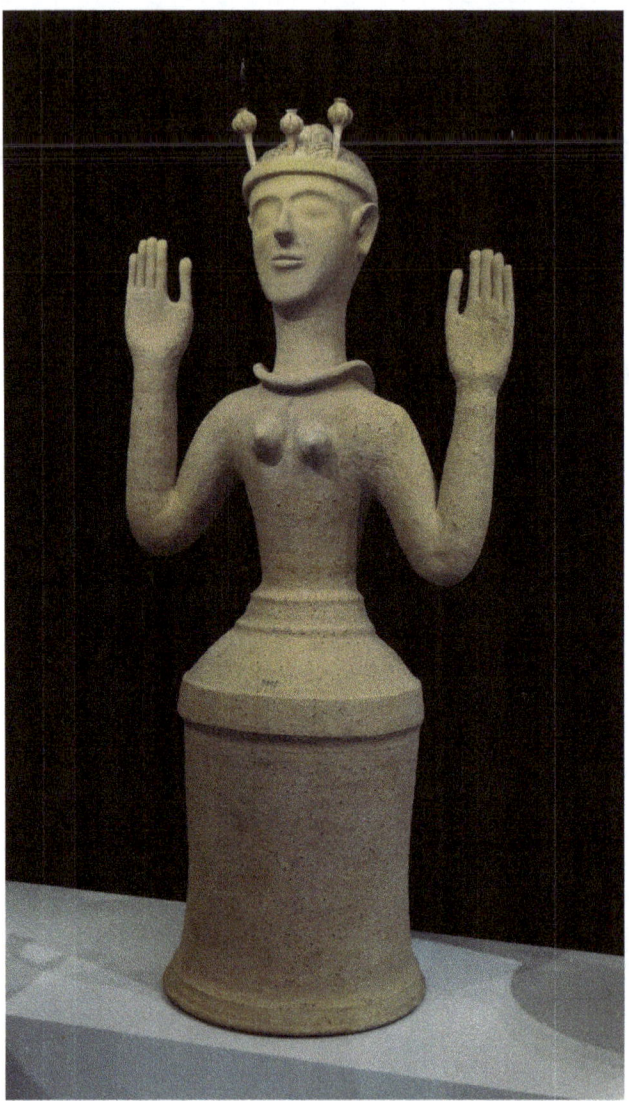

The Minoan Poppy Goddess is so-called because of the three poppy heads emerging from her crown.

She has also been described as praying, giving a greeting, a blessing, or a gesture of epiphany, symbolising her appearance in this world before humankind, or symbolising a divine revelation or inspiration.

Rather than being a cult image or a devotional image that is worshipped or venerated, her appearance in public sanctuaries suggests that this figurine, and others like it, is a votive offering left by devotees in a sacred place for spiritual purposes.

Figurines like this one have been dated to around 1400-1100 BCE, and have been found on Crete at Gazi, Knossos, Gournia, Myrtos, Gortys, and Prinias.

As a goddess, it is thought that she is a personification or a bringer of sleep or death, a symbolic connection with poppies that would continue into Greek and later Roman mythology.

The Assyrians were believed to have referred to poppy juice as '*aratpa-pal*', which has been speculated as possibly where the Latin word '*papaver*' evolved from, however there are no lexical sources for this in the field of Assyriology and this may be another misinterpretation of a Sumerian term. In the city of Nimrud, in the northwest palace of King Ashurnasirpal II (883-859 BCE), a series of bas-reliefs were found depicting a winged genie, holding what looks like a poppy plant with several poppy heads. They could also just as easily be pomegranates or lotus seed pods.

It is tempting to map these iconic images together and conclude that the poppy was seen as a gift from the gods, symbolising the divine, and those pictured with poppies were divinely appointed, protected by or acting on behalf of the divine, perhaps offering medicine, death, or a combination of all of these.

This is all purely speculative of course, looking back at a period of time through the lens of the Greek and Roman mythology which followed it, where such mythological associations are well documented and live on in modern culture to this day. As far as Egypt is concerned however, there is "*no archaeological confirmation of the plant in Egypt before the Ptolemaic period*" (305 BCE to 30 BCE).[4]

---

[4] Sinclair, A. [Forthcoming, late 2021]. High Times in Ancient Egypt: The Use and Abuse of Psychoactive Plant Identifications in Alternative / Pseudo-Egyptology.

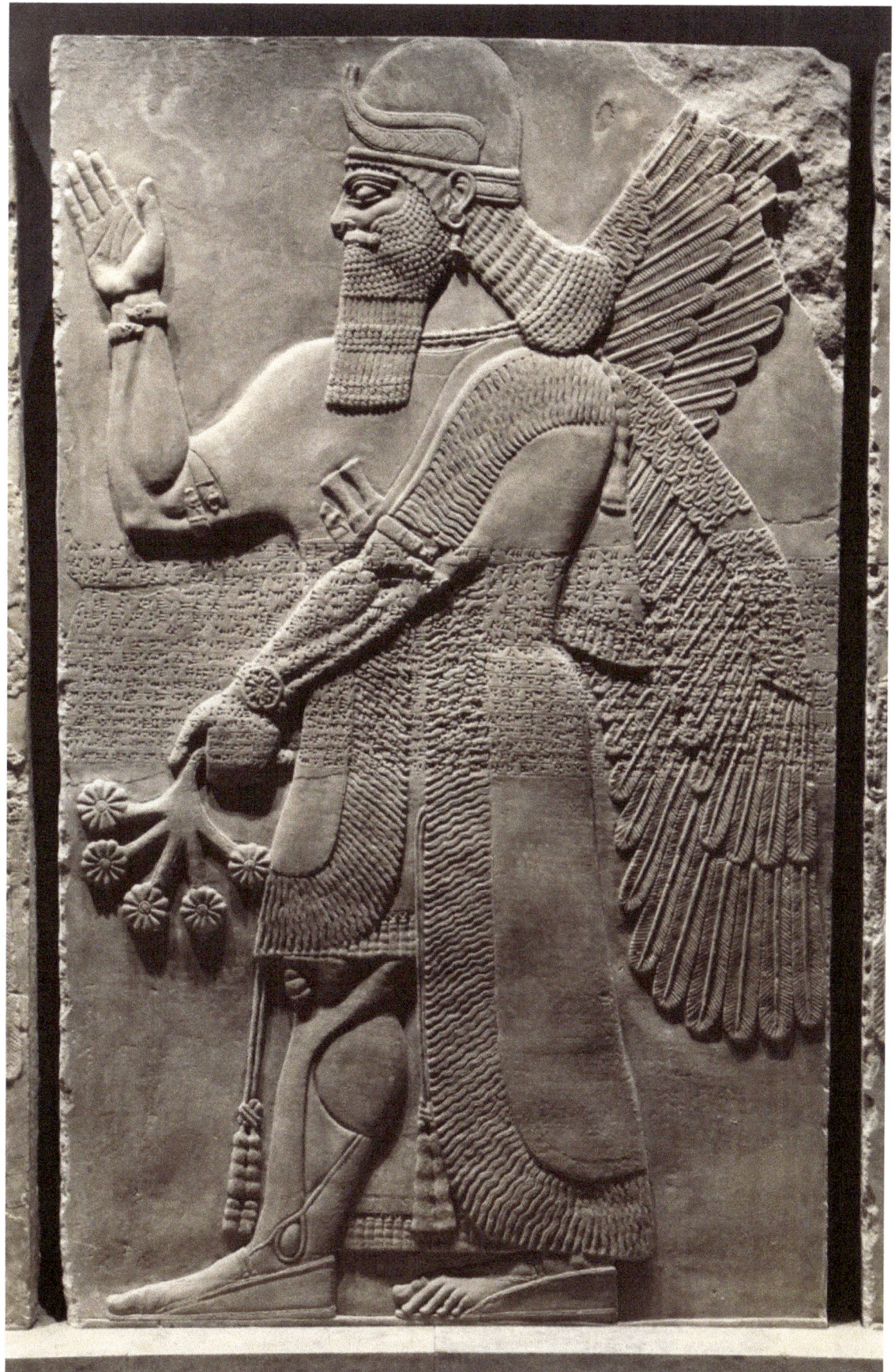
A winged bearded genie, Northwest palace of King Assurnasirpal II, Nimrud, c870 BCE

2. Antiquity: *Dark Mythology and the Light of Science (800 BCE-476 CE)*

2.1 Dark Mythology

The Ancient Greeks and Romans had shared beliefs about the origins of the world, and the forces of nature that affected their lives. These forces were personified in the form of deities and other figures. Although these deities may have had different names, their complex stories, family trees, motivations, and character traits were recognised as being equivalent, through the lens of '*Interpretatio Graeca*' (Interpretation by Greek models). They are woven into the overall telling of events that took place long before the creation of humankind. Of particular interest in Greek and Roman mythology there is a branch of the family tree of deities that represents darkness, trance, sleep, dreams, and death. They are often associated with or depicted as either holding poppies or wearing them. Perhaps the two best examples of this branch of the family tree to compare are based on the descriptions in Hesiod's '*Theogony*' and Ovid's '*Metamorphoses*' (Roman names are given in brackets where applicable).

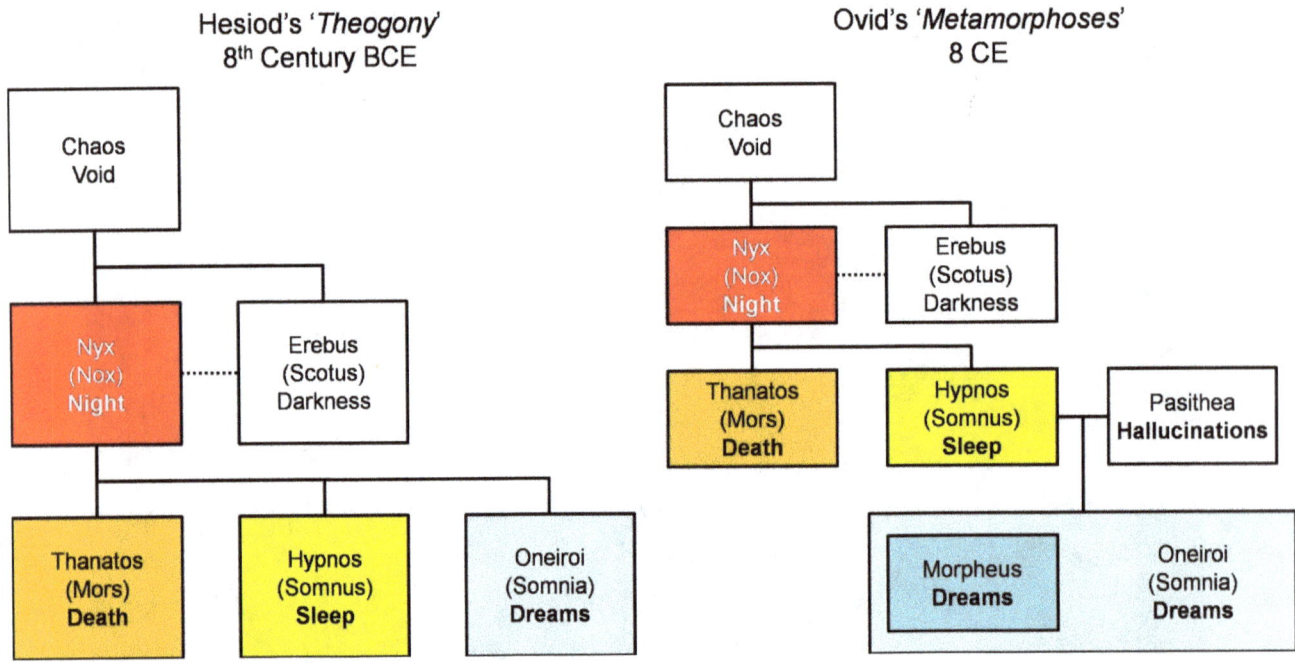

In Hesiod's '*Theogony*' the Oneiroi (*Somnia*) are the offspring of Nyx. In Ovid's '*Metamorphoses*', the Oneiroi are the offspring of Hypnos and Pasithea, including Morpheus who is the leader of the Oneiroi. These are the deities that bring us night, darkness, death, sleep, dreams, and hallucinations.

Many of the words relevant to this subject that we know today originated from Ancient Greek, and in some cases by their Latinisation, Latin equivalent, and sometimes by the adoption of Latin and Greek words into Old French and then into Middle English. For example:

Greek	Greek	Latin	Late Middle English
Opós (ὀπός)	*Ópion* (ὄπιον)	opium	opium
juice	poppy juice		

Nyx (*Nox*)

The Goddess of the night, born of Chaos, a shadowy figure with her shroud of darkness, she has enormous power, including the power to bring sleep or death Even the Olympian king of the gods Zeus (*Jupiter*) fears her.

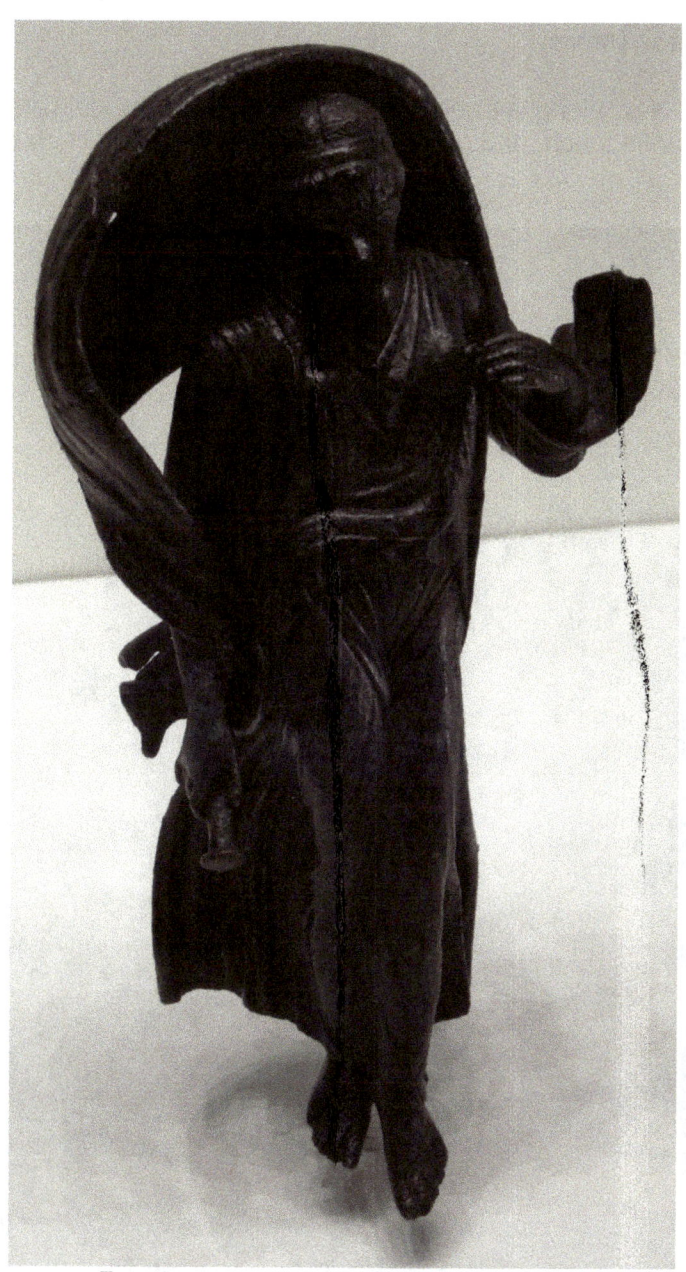

Roman bronze statuette of Nyx (*Nox*)
1st Century BCE

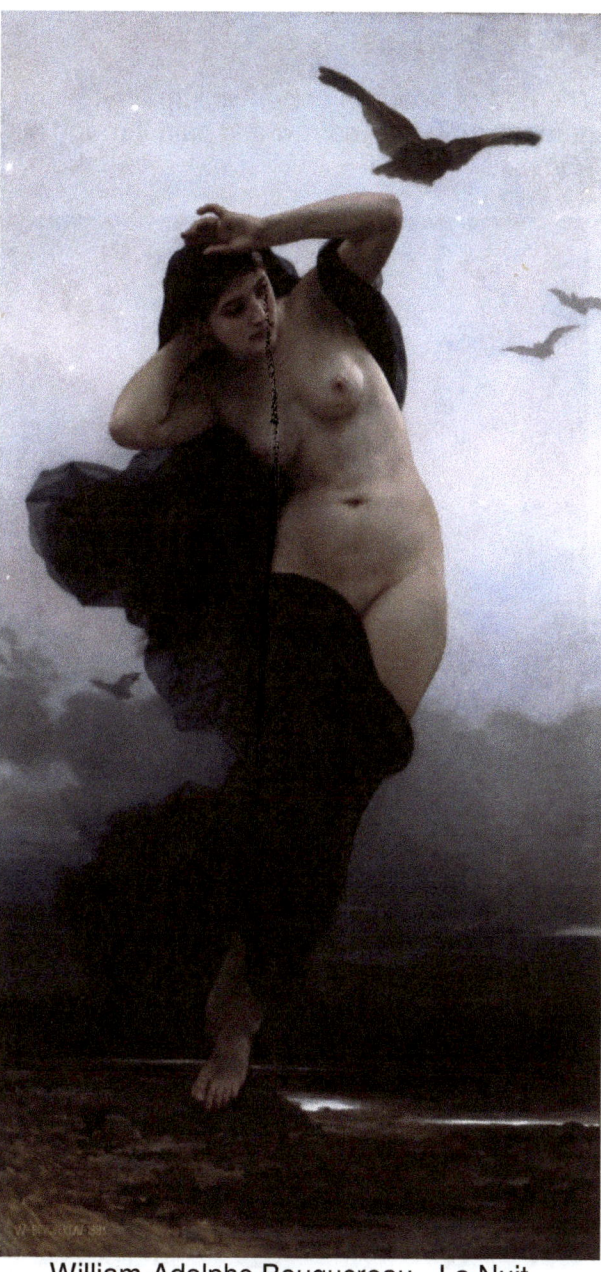

William-Adolphe Bouguereau - La Nuit
1883

Hypnos (*Somnus*)

The god of sleep, son of Nyx, his name is the origin of the word hypnosis. He and his brother Thanatos (*Mors*) live in the underworld Hades (*Orcus*), in caves next to each other which receive no sunlight or moonlight, and are completely silent. The caves are surrounded by poppies.

Thanatos (*Mors*)

The god of peaceful or non-violent death, son of Nyx, along with his twin brother Hypnos, he delivers humans from their sorrow and pain through his gentle touch, and brings them to the underworld Hades (*Orcus*).

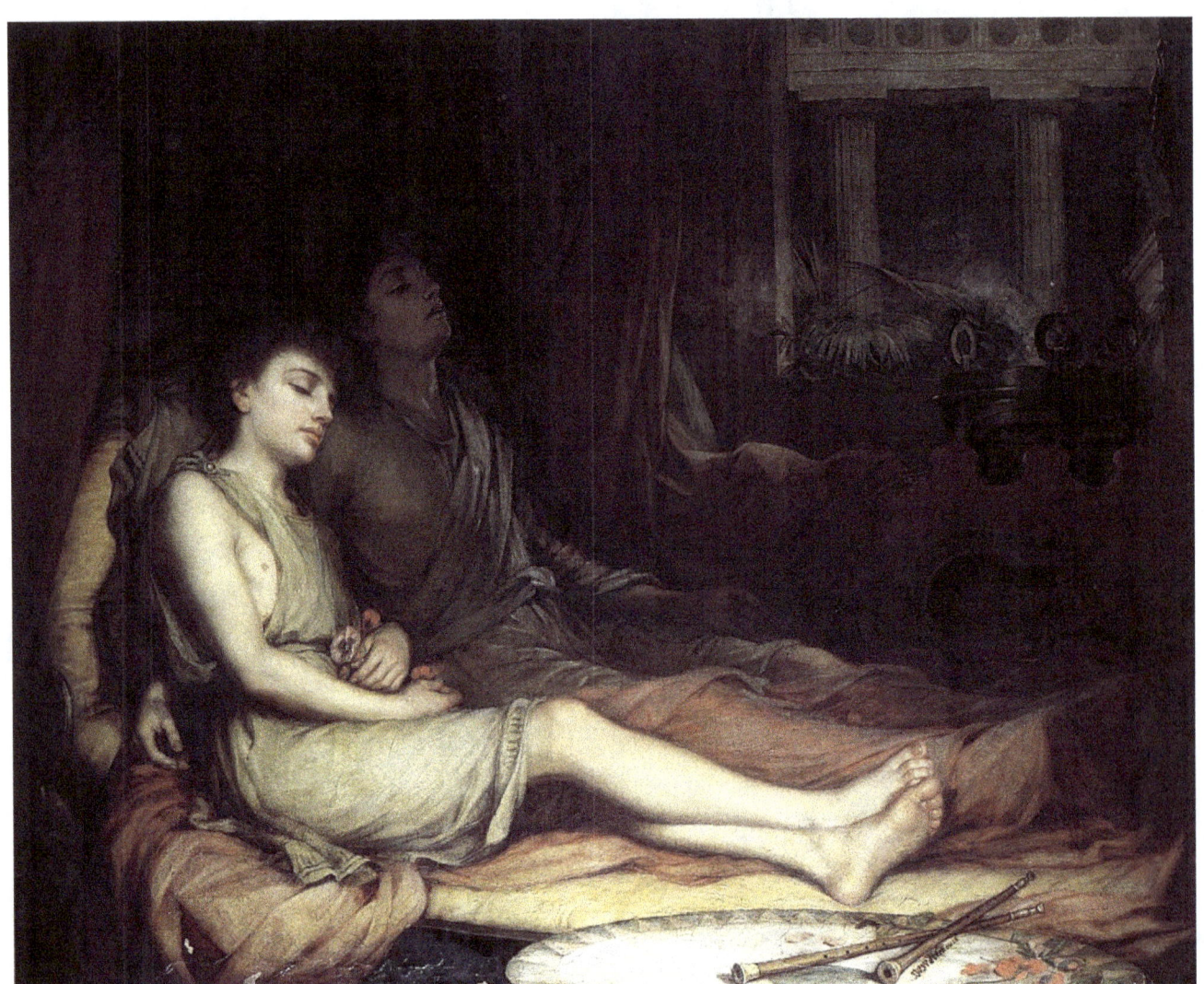

John William Waterhouse - Sleep and his half-brother Death, 1874

Note: Hypnos (*Somnus*) on the left is holding poppies under his left hand, and there are also poppies in the foreground on the bottom right. Thanatos (*Mors*) is pictured darker and in the shadows.

Morpheus

The god of dreams, son of Hypnos and Pasithea, his name is the origin of the word Morphine. He shapes and forms the dreams in which he can appear in any form as a messenger of the gods. He is one of the thousand sons of Hypnos, dream spirits called Oneiroi (*Somnia*), of which he is the leader.

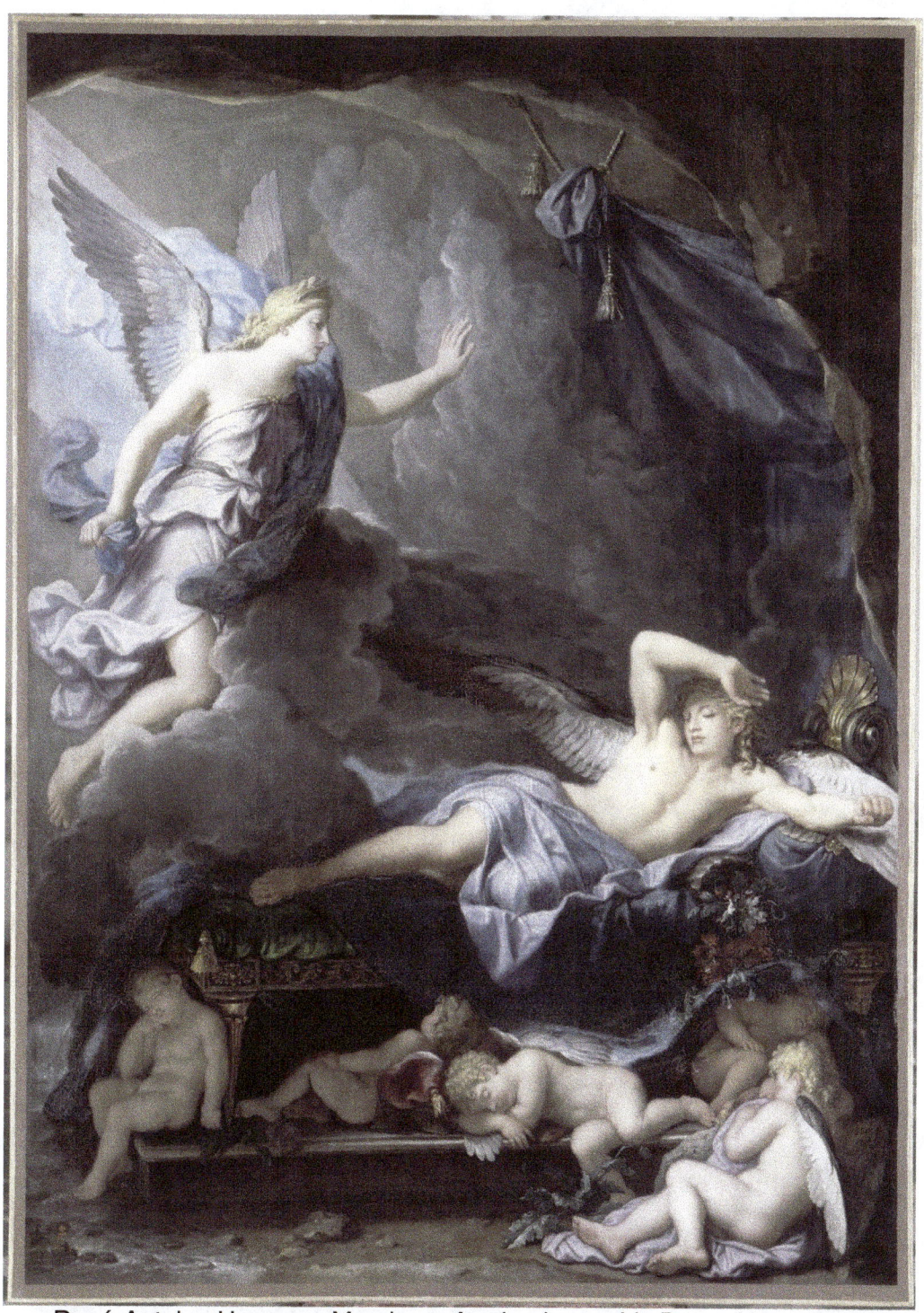

René-Antoine Houasse, Morpheus Awakening as Iris Draws Near, 1690

Note: In the foreground, below Morpheus are a bunch of poppies in various colours and states of blooming, and poppies in between two figures on the ground, Oneiroi (*Somnia*).

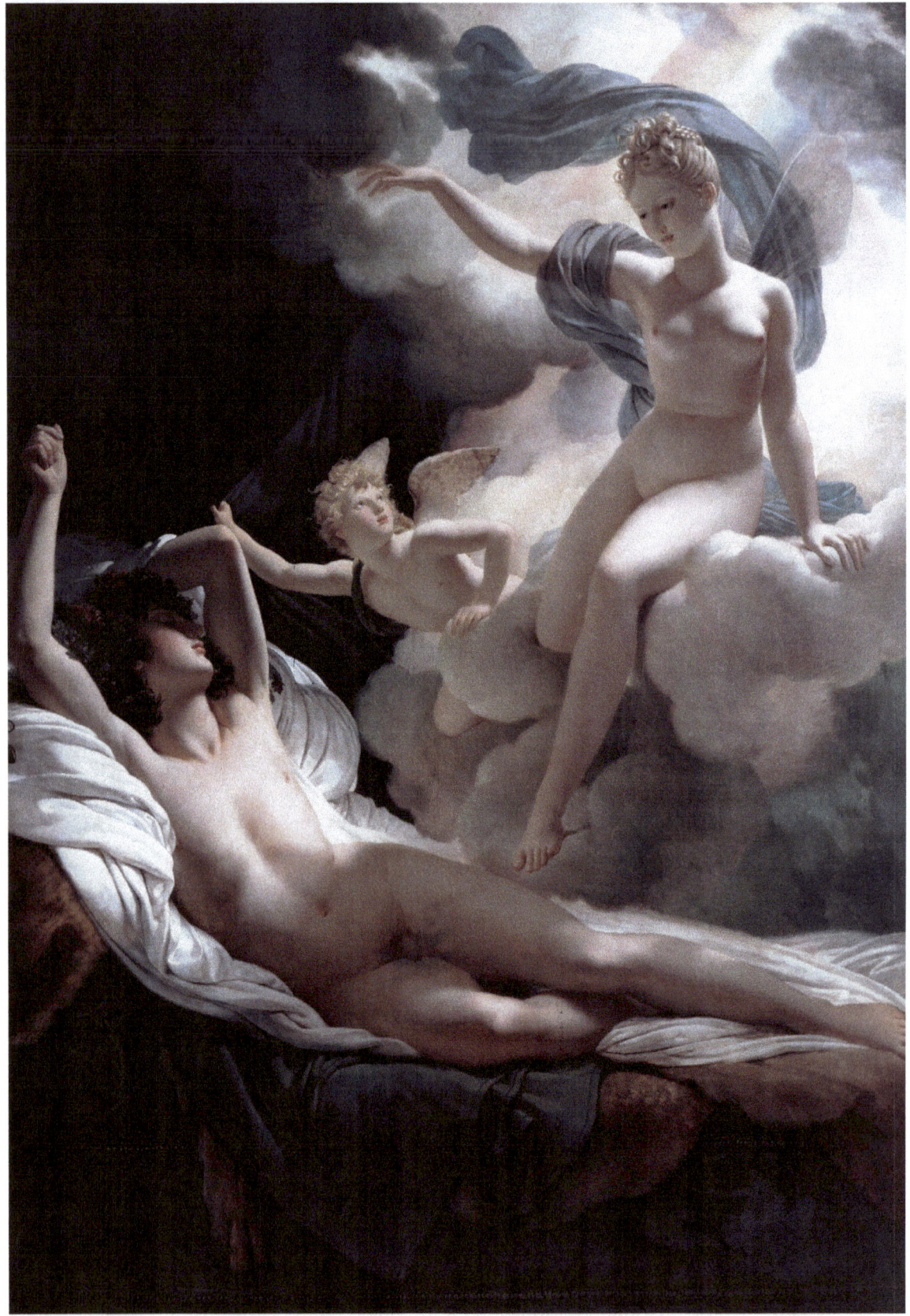

Guerin Pierre Narcisse, Morpheus and Iris, 1811

Note: Morpheus has a wreath of poppies around his head.

Pasithea

She is one of the Charites (*Gratiae*), she is the personification of relaxation, meditation, hallucinations, and altered states of consciousness. Queen of the Olympians Hera (*Juno*) offers her hand in marriage to Hypnos in return for a favour.

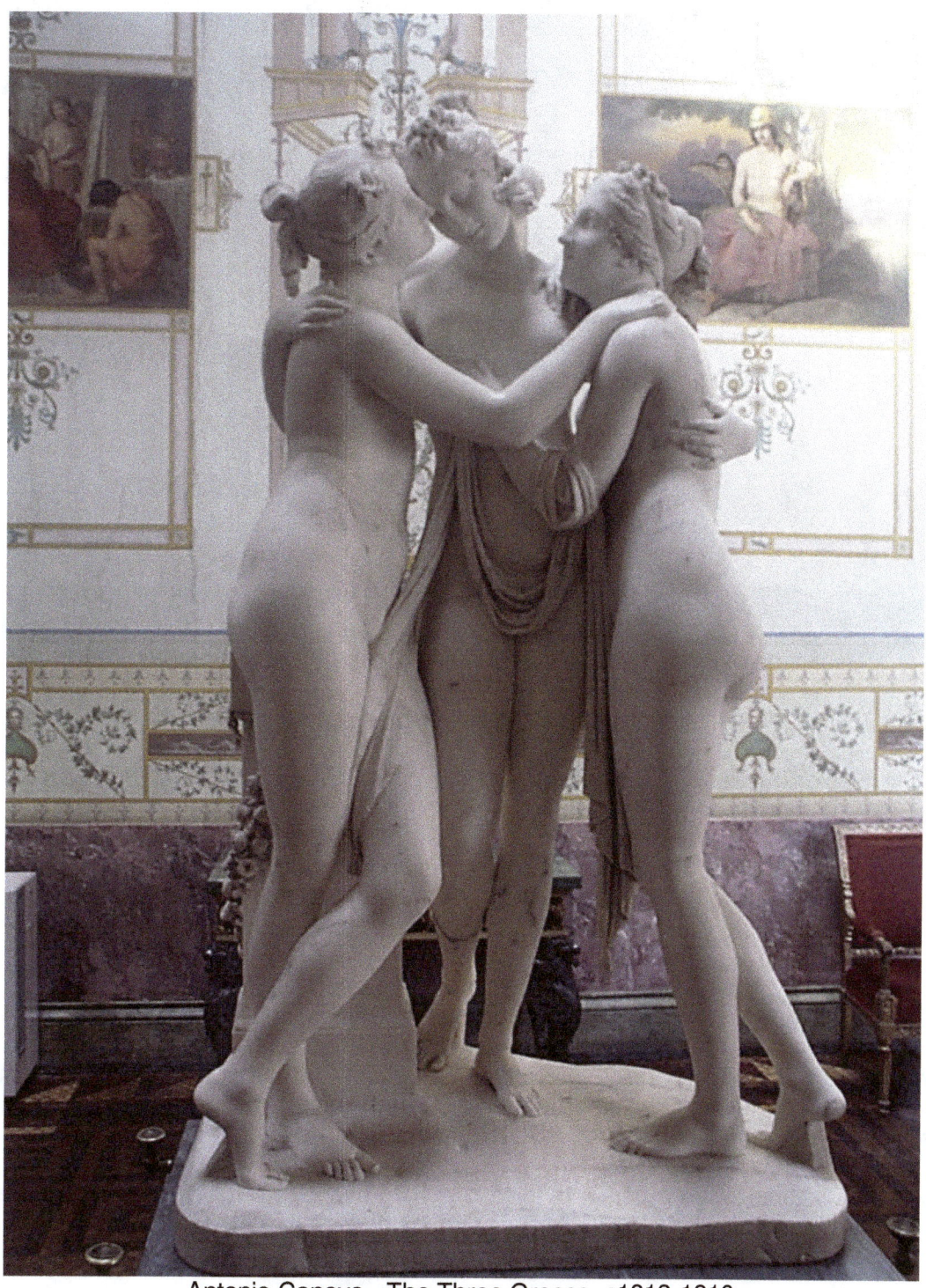

Antonio Canova - The Three Graces, c1813-1816

Note: Pasithea is possibly the figure on the left, with flowers behind her that could be interpreted as poppies.

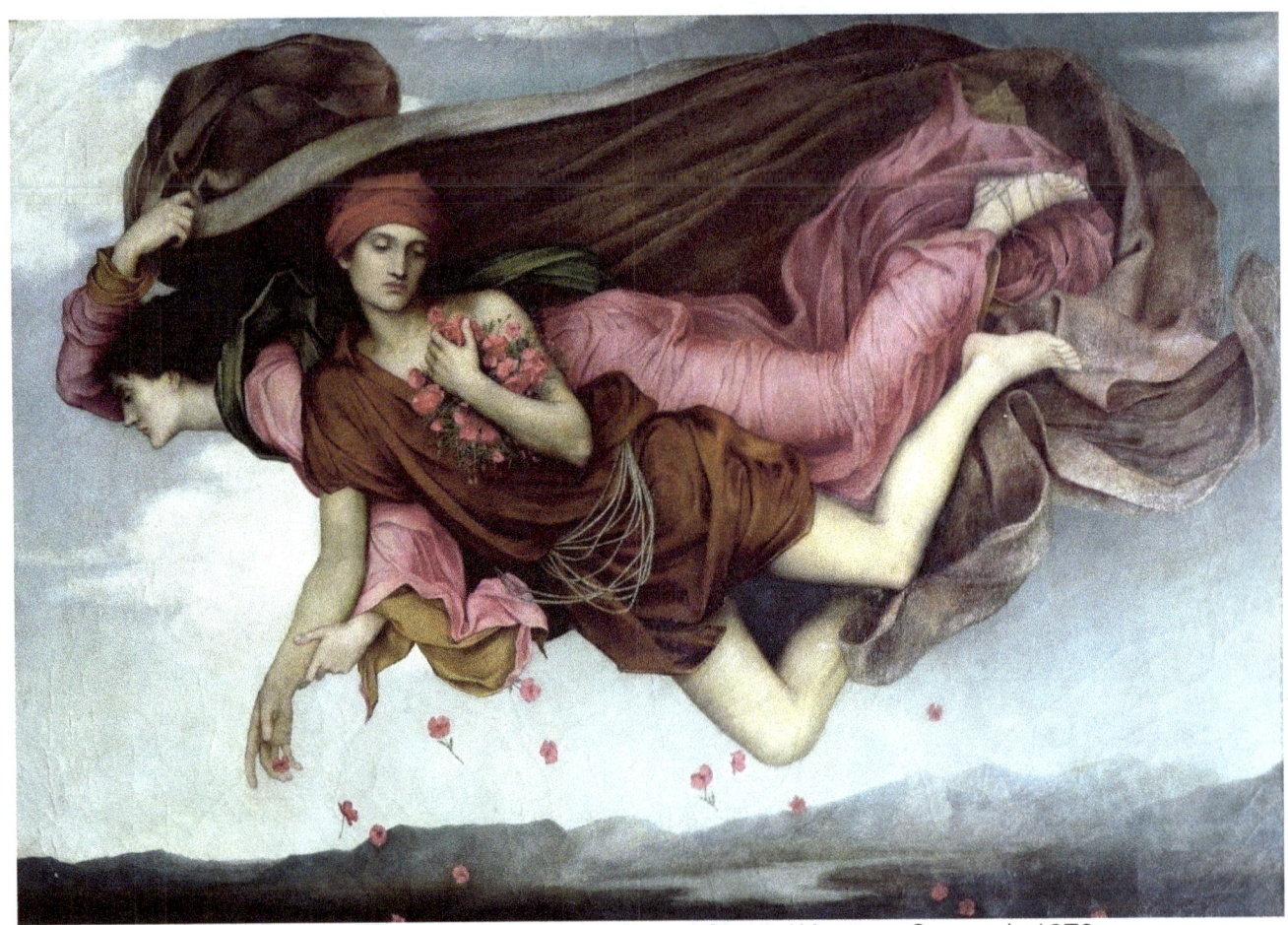

Evelyn de Morgan, Night (Nyx, *Nox*) and Sleep (*Hypnos, Somnus*), 1878

Note: Hypnos (Somnus) is scattering poppies as Nyx (Nox) is darkening the sky

According to Hesiod there was a city near Corinth called '*Mekonê*' (city of poppies). This city is believed to have earned its name from the cultivation of poppies in this area.

Homer writes in his 'Odyssey' that Helen of Troy serves opium dissolved in wine as a potion to cause "forgetfulness of evil". Apollonius of Rhodes writes in the 'Argonautica' that the poppy grows in the the botanical garden belonging to Hekatê (*Trivia*), the goddess of crossways, magic and witchcraft, near Kolchis.

This is also the place where the goddess of agriculture Demeter (*Ceres*) discovered the fruit of the poppy, and in despair over the seizure of her daughter Persephone (*Proserpina*) by the ruler of the underworld Pluto, she ate the poppies in order to fall asleep and forget her grief. As a result of this, Demeter (*Ceres*) is sometimes depicted or described as holding a small bouquet of poppies in one arm as well as wheat in the other.

The Eleusinian Mysteries were a series of initiations held every year for the cult of Demeter (Ceres) and Persephone (Proserpina) in Eleusis, Ancient Greece, later spreading to Ancient Rome.

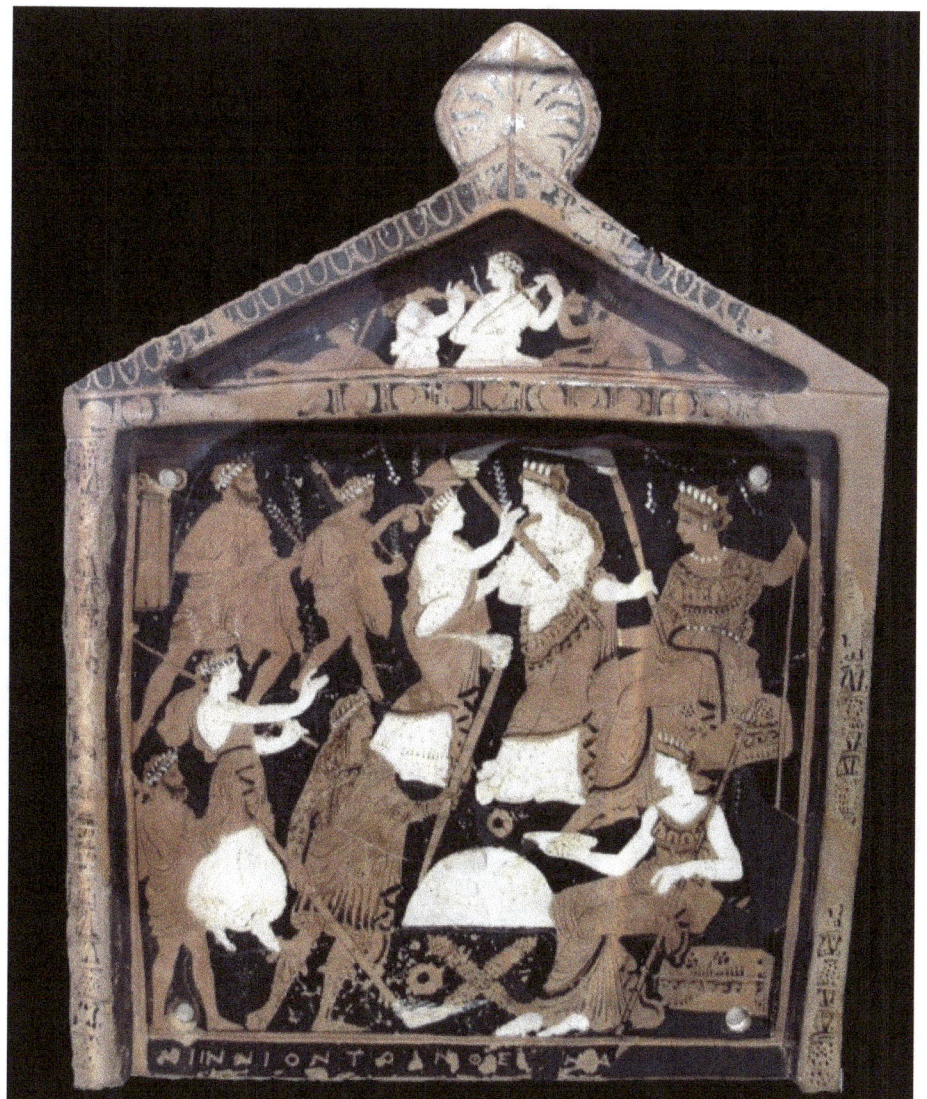

A votive plaque depicting Eleusinian Mysteries, by an artist called Ninion, c4th century BCE

Note: There appear to be two poppies depicted in the foreground, and some wheat, and several people are holding drinking vessels, suggesting the drinking of some kind of ritualised concoction. The temporary hypnotic and narcotic effects of opium consumed in such cult or religious rituals would have given a powerful and symbolic mind-altering representation of death and the descent into the underworld, and then an ascent from the underworld into rebirth, transmigration of the soul, reincarnation, and reunion.

2.2 The Light of Science

There are accounts from ancient Greece that opium was consumed in several ways, by inhalation of vapours, suppositories, medical ointments applied to the skin, or concocted with hemlock for suicide (also known as '*the Keian custom*', or a kind of voluntary euthanasia).

Hippocrates (c460-370 BCE) is referred to as the 'Father of Medicine' because of his contributions to the field which revolutionised ancient Greek medicine. In the Corpus Hippocraticum there are references to the poppy and its use in medicine, distinguishing different types of poppy, including white, fire-red, and black varieties, and poppy juice as a hypnotic and narcotic, and the nutrition provided by poppy seeds. He also refers to the opium poppy as sleep-inducing.

Between 336 and 323 BCE Alexander the Great launched a prolonged military campaign of conquest against the Achaemenid Persian Empire of King Darius III, continuing on as far east as India.

It is believed that he brought opium thebaicum with him as medicine for his soldiers, and that subsequently knowledge of cultivation and production of opium spread in the regions that his armies conquered. However it is also likely that these regions already had this knowledge as a result of trade in the Achaemenid Empire as far back as 500 BCE or even further.

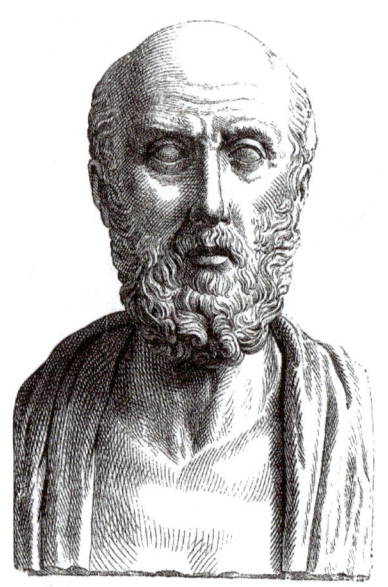

An engraving of a bust of Hippocrates, 1881

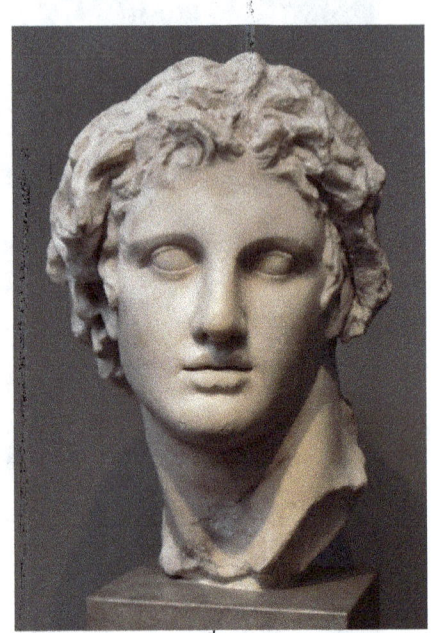

A Roman copy of 3rd Century BCE bust of Alexander the Great

Pliny the Elder (c23-79 CE) was a Roman author, naturalist, natural philosopher, and a naval and army commander of the Roman Empire, even known to the emperor Vespasian.

His '*Naturalis Historia*' mentions the poppy in book 20, notably the heraclium poppy being "pounded in a mortar for epilepsy", and served in an *acetabulum* (a form of bowl) with white wine to avoid the possibility of vomiting. References to opium being served dissolved into wine are commonplace after this point.

"decoquitur et bibitur contra vigilias, eademque aqua fovent ora. optimum in siccis et ubi raro pluat.

"boiled and drunk against insomnia. The same water is used for the face. The best in dry conditions where rain is rare.

Cum capita ipsa et folia decocuntur, sucus meconium vocatur multum opio ignavior".

With the heads themselves and leaves are boiled, juice is called meconium and is a lot less potent than opium".

Pedanius Dioscorides (c40-90 CE) was a Greek pharmacologist, botanist, and physician in the Roman Army. His work '*De Materia Medica*' gives a detailed description of medicinal uses of plants, including the poppies '*Mekon Agrios*' and '*Mekon Emeros*' which cause sleep, and can be used to treat inflammation, boiled with honey to make a cough mixture. He does however bluntly warn that too much of it can kill.

"A little of it (taken with as much as a grain of ervum) is a pain-easer, a sleep-causer, and a digester, helping coughs and abdominal cavity afflictions.

Taken as a drink too often it hurts (making men lethargic) and it kills. It is helpful for aches, sprinkled on with rosaceum; and for pain in the ears dropped in them with oil of almonds, saffron, and myrrh.

For inflammation of the eyes it is used with a roasted egg yolk and saffron, and for erysipela and wounds with vinegar; but for gout with women's milk and saffron.

Put up with the finger as a suppository it causes sleep".

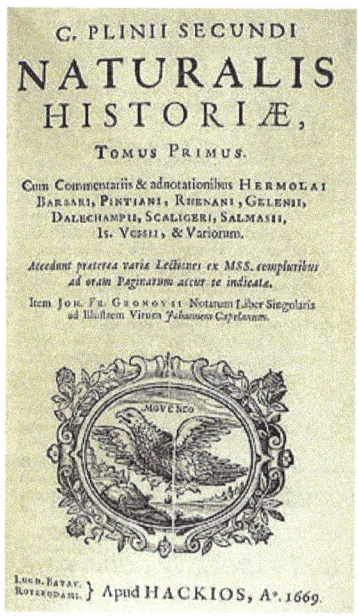
A 1669 edition of Pliny the Elder's *'Naturalis Historia'*

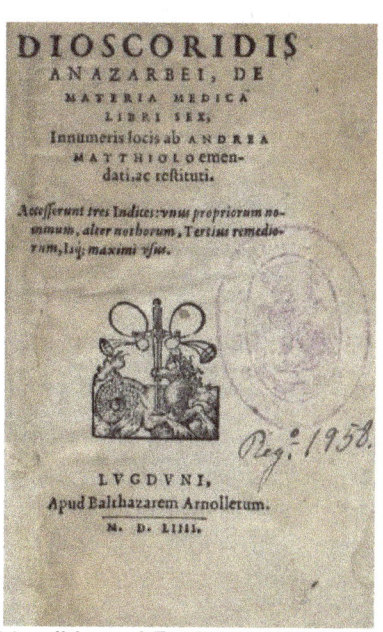
A 1554 edition of Pedanius Dioscorides's *'De Materia Medica'*

The word '*Mekonion*' and its Latin version '*Meconium*' was later used as a kind of nickname to describe the first excreta of a newly born infant, composed of materials ingested during the time the infant spends in the womb, on account of its raw opium tar-like appearance.

Greek	Greek	Latin	Early Modern English, c1706
mḗkōn (μήκων)	mēkṓnion (μηκώνιον)	mēcōnium	meconium
poppy	poppy juice	poppy juice	poppy juice

Aulus Cornelius Celsus (c25 BCE-50 CE) was a Roman encyclopaedist who gathered together medical knowledge in his '*De Medicina*':

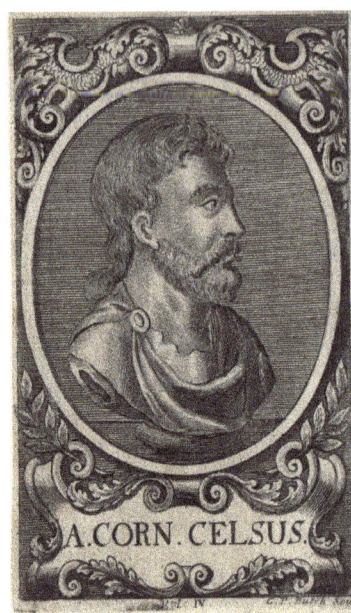

A portrait of Aulus Cornelius Celsus by Geog Paul Busch, 1719

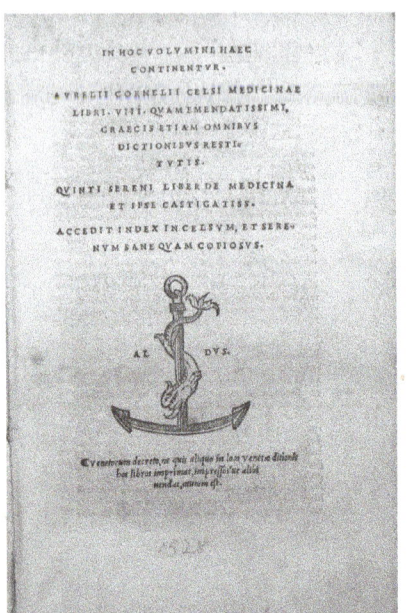

A 1528 edition of Celsus's '*De Medicina*'

"Somno vero aptum est papaver, lactuca, maximeque aestiva, cuius coliculus iam lacte repletus est, morum, porrus. Sensus excitat nepeta, thymum, satureia, hysopum, praecipueque puleium, ruta et cepe".

"Sleep however apt is the poppy, lettuce, mostly in summer, whose stalk already with milkiness is replete, mulberry. Senses excited by: catmint, thyme, savoury, hyssop, and especially pennyroyal, rue and onion".

Scribonius Largus (c1-50 CE) was the court physician to the Roman emperor Claudius, during which time he compiled over 200 medical prescriptions in '*De compositione medicamentorum liver*', relying heavily on his tutors, friends, and the writings of eminent physicians, and also including traditional remedies. A large part of this work formed the basis of '*De Medicamentes Empiricis Physicis, et Rationibus*' by Marcellus Empiricus in around 410 CE.

"Sed opium et in hoc et in omni collyrio medicamentoque verum adicere oportet, quod ex lacte ipso silvatici papaveris capitum fit, non ex suco foliorum eius".

"But opium and in this and all eye ointments and medicine it is necessary to add in this, which out of milk itself wild poppy head is made, not out of juice from its leaves".

Galen (129-210 CE) was a Greek physician and philosopher of the Roman Empire, and considered one of the greatest medical researchers of antiquity who wrote some fourteen books on the method of medicine.

He is also credited with having popularised the prescription of opium based remedies across the Roman world, and for having prescribed opium to Emperor Marcus Aurelius for chest and stomach conditions.

Marcus Aurelius apparently disliked its hypnotic and narcotic effects, and stopped taking it, but then found he was no longer able to sleep, so began taking it again. This is often cited as one of the first examples of addiction to opium.

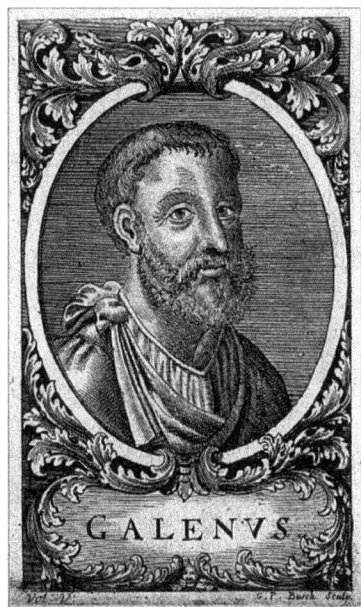

An 18th century portrait of Galen by Georg Paul Busch

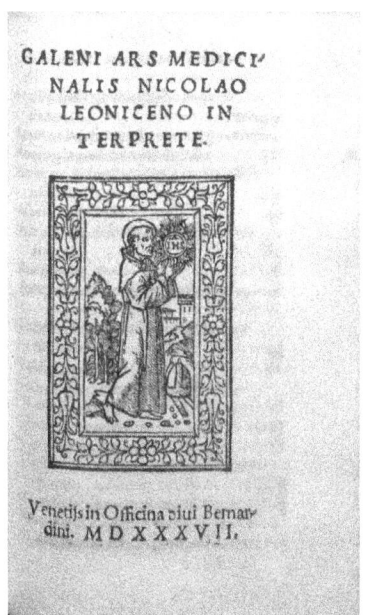

A 1537 edition of Galen's '*Ars Medicinalis*'

As well as being dissolved into wine, opium was also prepared as a bitter tea called 'cretic wine', or even available dried and pressed into tablets which were available in specialist stalls in most marketplaces.

Roman soldiers who began construction on the Antonine Wall in 142 CE (from the Firth of Forth and the Firth of Clyde in what is today the central belt of Scotland) are known to have imported opium and wine among their supplies, perhaps medicinally to treat whipworm, round worm, and fleas, and perhaps also recreationally to dull the misery of the cold and wet weather so far north at the edge of the known world.

3. The Middle Ages: *East-West Exchange (476-1453)*

When the Western Roman Empire collapsed in 476 CE, much of the manufacture, trade, architecture, literacy, law, and international language of science and literature was lost in Western Europe. The Eastern Roman Empire, which became known as the Byzantine Empire, continued and preserved these important medical works, which were then studied and translated into Greek and later Arabic.

By the early Middle Ages the 'Silk Road' was already a long and well established trade route between East and West, and was central to the economy, culture, and politics. The name 'Silk Road' comes from the profitable trade in silk from China.

As well as silk and other luxury items, many other exchanges took place simultaneously in the form of cultural trade, religions, philosophies, sciences, and technologies like paper and gunpowder.

The word 'road' suggests land, but there were also well established routes by sea described as the maritime branch or the 'sea road'. Perhaps because of favourable sea routes and geographic location, it was Arab traders who introduced opium to India and China between 400 and 700 CE.

From the 8th Century there was a period of cultural, economic, and scientific flourishing that was later referred to as the 'Islamic Golden Age'. This started with the Abbasid caliphate and the building of the House of Wisdom in Baghdad, which was the world's largest city at the time. Scholars and polymaths from different parts of the world were tasked with gathering together all of the world's knowledge and translating it into Syriac and Arabic.

Rhazes (854-932), the Persian physician and alchemist, was born in the city of Ray (Shahr-e Rey) on the Great Silk Road. He studied medical texts from both Islamic writers and Greek writers, particularly Galen.

He is the first Arabic-writing physician to make thorough use of Hippocrates's writings as a basis for his own medical system.

His most important work is '*Kitab al-Hawi fi al-tibb*' (The comprehensive book of medicine), containing medical notes taken throughout his career, extracts of all of his sources with observations from his own experience, including the use of opium for melancholy, diseases of the intestines, the eyes, painful joints and gout:

> "*Where gout is accompanied by high fever, the recipe contains seeds that cause diuresis without giving out much heat, such as those of white colchicum, water melon and cucumber. These, in equal parts, are mixed with one third of a part of opium, and an oral dose of four dirhams (12 g) of the mixture with the same amount of sugar is analgesic and effective within the hour*".

> "*Where there is no high fever, the ingredients, in an oral remedy, are: colchicum, opium, borax, colocynth, ammi, aristolochia, and mountain thyme*".

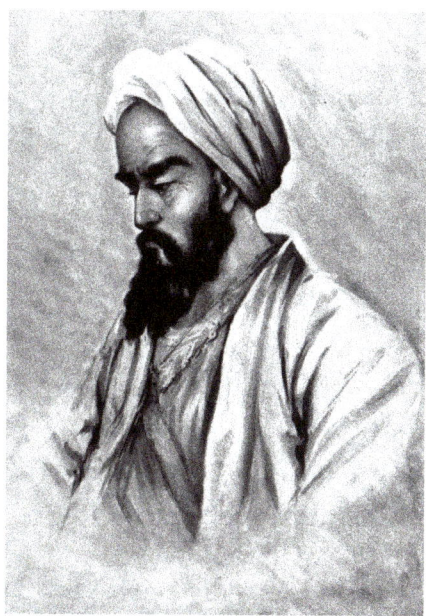
A Portrait of Rhazes

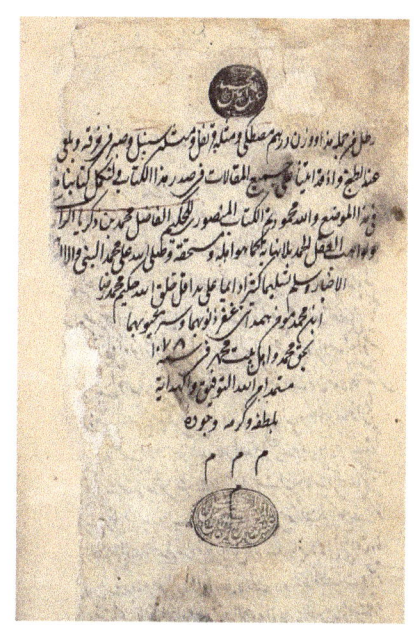
Rhaze's 'The Comprehensive Book of Medicine'

Abulcasis (936-1013) was an Arab Andalusian physician, surgeon, and chemist, described as 'the father of modern surgery'. His work '*Kitab al-Tasrif*' contains information about illnesses, treatments and surgical procedures. Translated into Latin in the 1100s, it gives an account of the use of opium and mandrake as surgical anaesthetic.

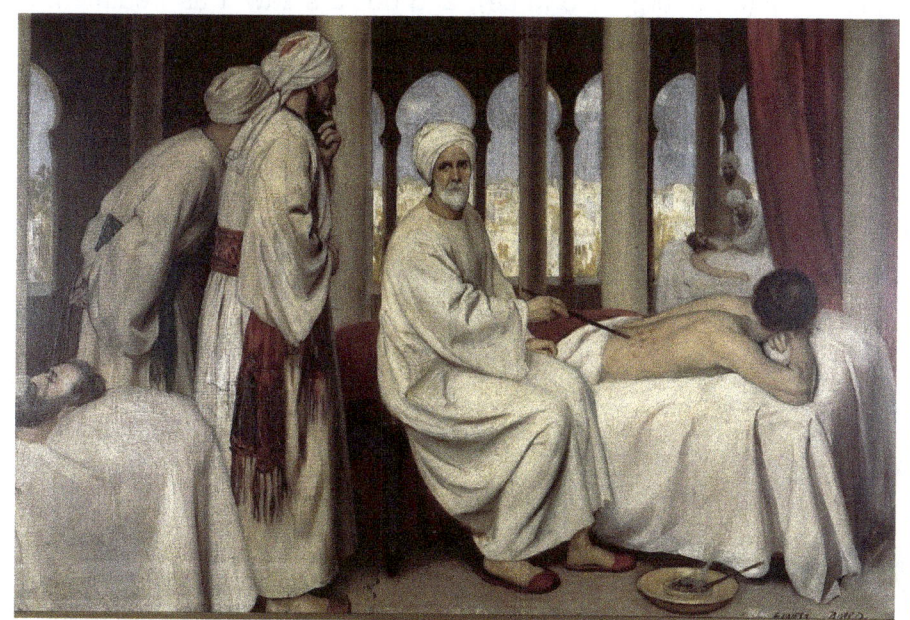
Albucasis blistering a patient in the hospital at Cordova, 1100

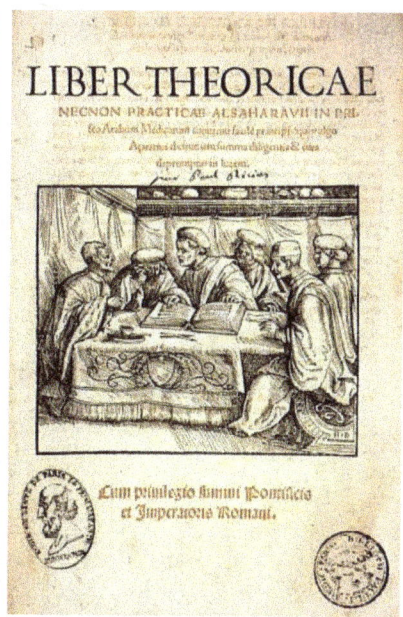
A Latin translation of Al-Zahrawi's Kitab al-Tasrif, 1541

Avicenna (980-1037) was a Persian physician. His influential '*Qanun-e dâr Tâb*' (The Canon of Medicine) mentions the poppy under '*Afion*' and describes in detail how opium can be used to treat any type of pain because of its strong analgesic and sedative properties, recommended for chronic headaches, joint pain, toothache, pain in the ears, with remedies by mouth, absorbed by the skin, rectally, or nasally.

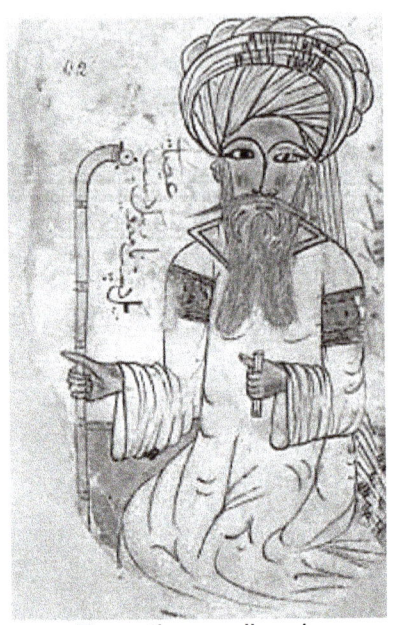

Avicenna. From the medieval manuscript 'Subtleties of Truth', 1271

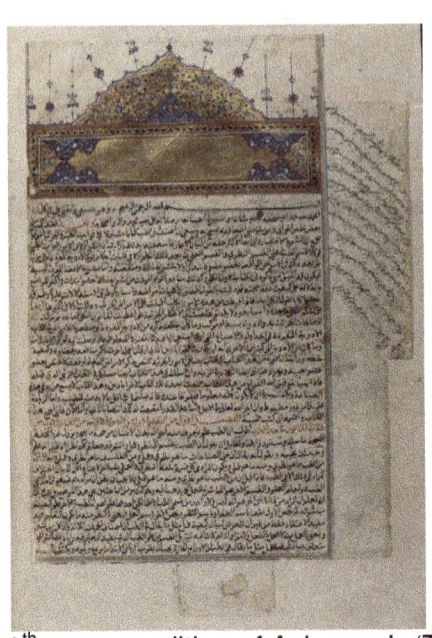

A 16th century edition of Avicenna's 'The Canon of Medicine'

Su Shi (Sū Shì, 1037-1101) also known as Su Dongpo (Sū Dōngpō) was a famous poet, writer, and politician of the Song Dynasty. He referred to the use of opium which was often given nicknames like yingsu soup or black spice.

Daoists believed that it could regulate *chi* (qì, energy, life force), and doctors saw it as treatment to regulate the digestive system and enhance sexual health and ability.

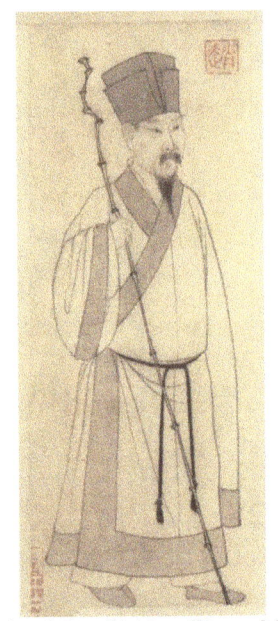

Portrait of Su Shi by Zhao Mengfu

道人劝饮鸡苏水

Dào rén quàn yǐn jī sū shuǐ

"Daoists often persuade you to drink the jisu water

童子能煎莺粟汤。

tóngzǐ néng jiān yīng sù tāng".

but even a child can prepare the yingsu soup".

During the Crusades in the Middle East between 1099 and 1291, the trade at this crossroads extended to Europe as well. Wool and textiles from northern Europe made their way to the Middle East and Asia, while silk, cotton, spices, oranges, and sugar made their way to Europe. It is possible that opium was also transported along these routes, and that soldiers returning home from the Crusades brought supplies of opium back with them.

The Byzantine Empire, centred around Constantinople (now Istanbul), became an important trading point between East and West, and opium produced in the fields of Anatolia found its way in both directions, and indeed into the court at Constantinople.

In the Islamic World there was an increase of opinion against the use of opium for recreational purposes, that it was unclean and un-Islamic.

Its use in medicine continued, and in the rituals of dervishes, who claimed that the drug bestowed them with visionary glimpses of future happiness.

Differences in theological beliefs between the Catholic and the Greek Orthodox Church caused a series of rifts and mistrust between East and West.

In the eyes of the Catholic Inquisition, everything from the East was characterised was wicked, evil, and linked to the devil, and opium, which had been very much associated with the East had become something of a taboo subject, and written records became scarce in Western Europe from this point.

4. Early Modern Times: *Renaissance (1453-1800)*

4.1 The Near East: The Ottoman World

On the 29th May 1453, the Ottoman forces under Mehmed II captured the city of Constantinople, thereby bringing about the end of the Byzantine Empire.

Greek scholars migrated to Italy with their texts and brought about a revival of interest in Greek and classical learning in general. The surviving texts were translated into Latin and printed using the latest technology.

Sabuncuoğlu Şerafeddin (1385-1468) was an Ottoman surgeon and physician. His book '*Cerrahiyyet'u"l Haniye*' (Imperial Medicine) described the use of opium to treat migraine headaches, sciatica, and other painful ailments.

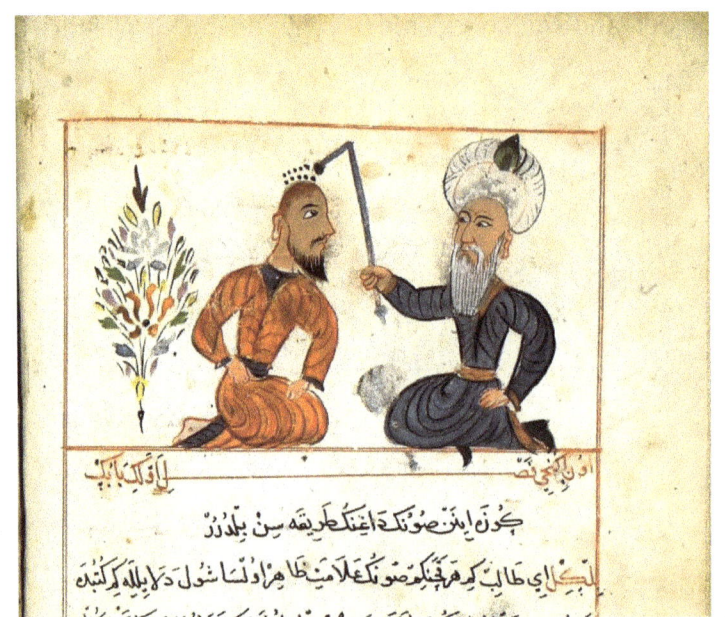

Sabuncuoğlu Şerafeddin's 'Imperial Medicine', 15th Century CE

By 1573 the recreational use of opium was continuing in the Ottoman Empire, according to the Venetian Costantino Garzoni in his text "Relazione dell'impero Ottomano del senatore Costantino Garzoni stato all'ambascieria di Costantinopoli nel 1573".

He states that many of the Turkish natives of Constantinople regularly drank:

> "[a] certain black water made with opium that makes them feel good, but to which they become so addicted, if they try to go without, they will quickly die".

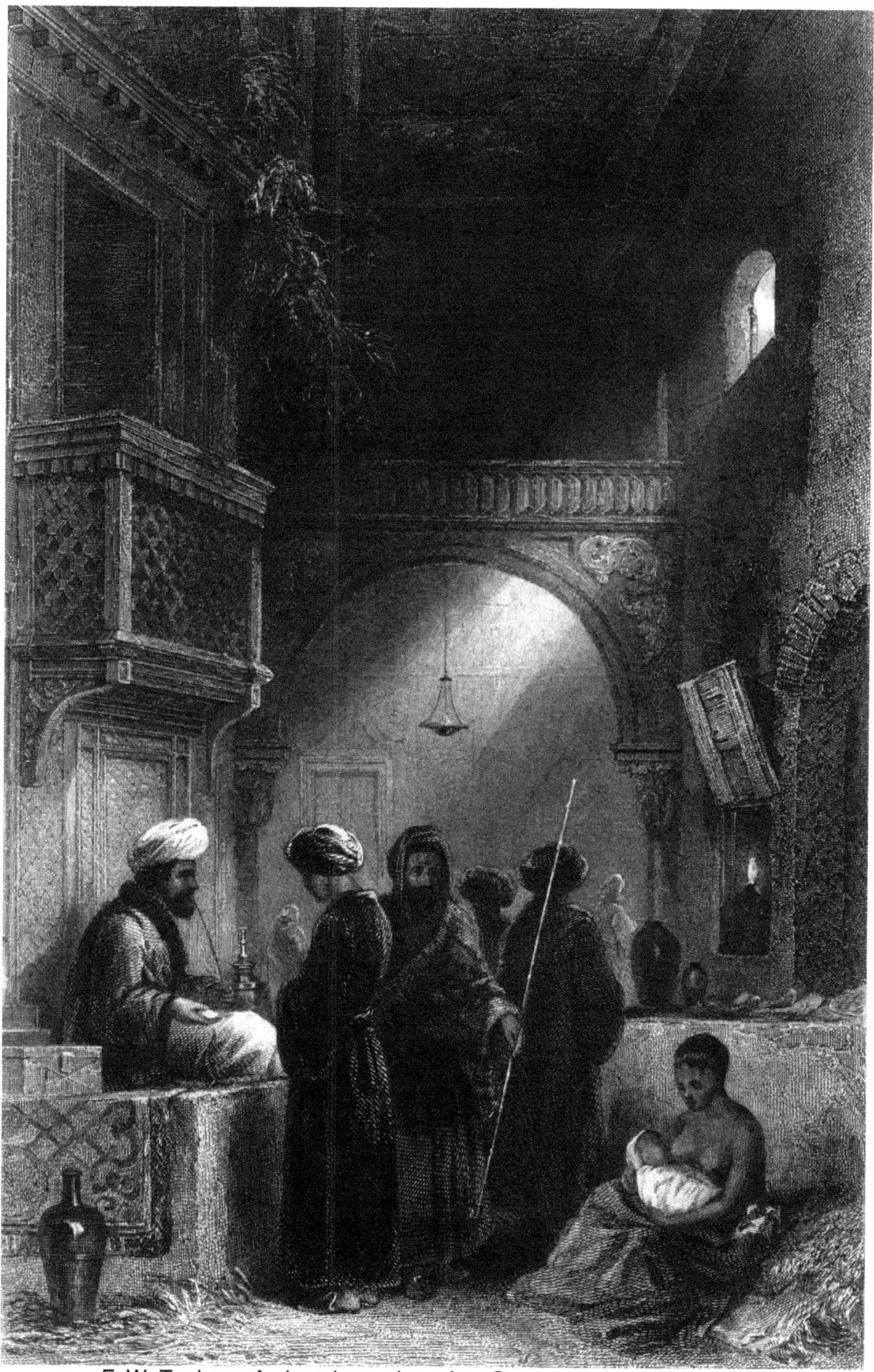
F. W. Topham, An imaginary view of an Ottoman opium seller c1850

4.2 The Far East: Chinese Dominance

In 1483 Xu Boling wrote the earliest clear description of the use of opium as a recreational drug, describing how the Ming dynasty Chenghua Emperor sent an expedition to procure opium at a price "equal to that of gold" in Hainan, Fujian, Zhejiang, Sichuan and Shaanxi, where it is close to the western lands of Xiyu.

Li Shizhen (1518-1593) was a Chinese physician who compiled 53 volumes worth of Chinese medicine called the 'Compendium of Materia Medica' in English. The traditional Chinese name 本草綱目 translates as 'Principles and Species of Roots and Herbs'. This renowned work includes the standard medical uses for opium, adding:

> *"It is mainly used to treat masculinity, strengthen sperm, and regain vigour. It enhances the art of alchemists, sex and court ladies. Frequent use helps to cure the chronic diarrhea that causes the loss of energy ... Its price equals that of gold".*

The first draft was completed in 1578, but it was not printed until after his death in 1593. Sadly, the Ming Dynasty emperor Wanli did not pay much attention to it.

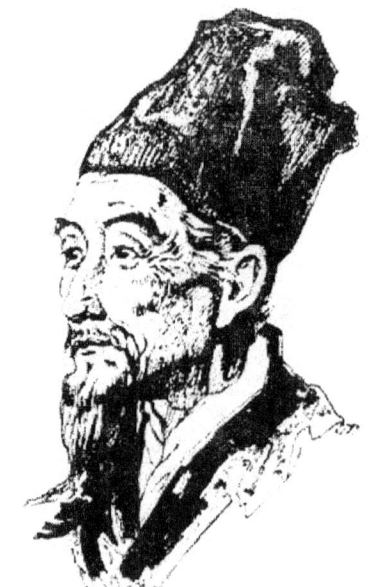
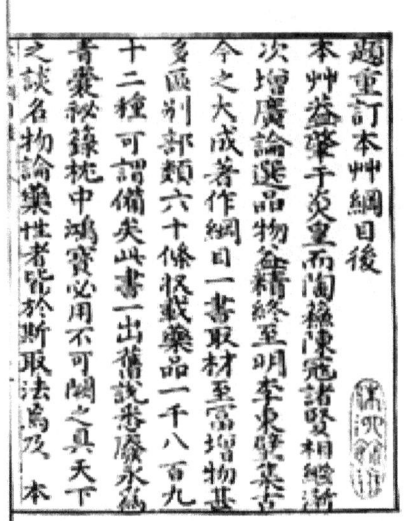
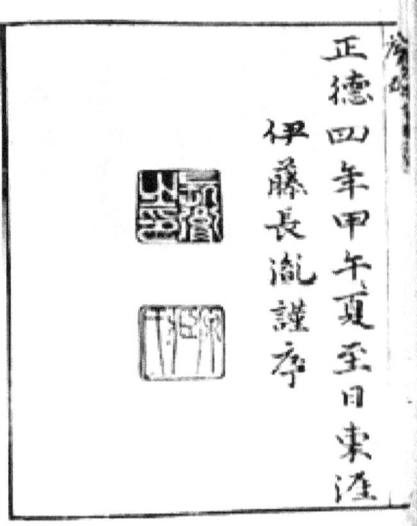

An Illustration of Li Shizhen   A 1593 edition of Li Shizen's 'Compendium of Materia Medica'

Ming Dynasty rulers of China received gifts of opium known as *wuxiang* or 'black spice' via a system of tribute, in which surrounding nations (Brunei, *Cambodia, Japan, Korea, Malaysia, Nepal, Philippines, Ryukyu, Siam, Tibet, Vietnam,* and *Ceylon*) would formally acknowledge China's superiority with an exchange of gifts, sometimes up to 100kg (220 lb) of opium, along with other exotic goods such as frankincense, ivory, and peacock feathers.

In 1639 Ming Emperor Chongzhen issued a national ban on tobacco, and added that tobacco addicts be executed. This was later expanded to include all those who possessed tobacco. The practice of smoking a mixture of tobacco and opium was replaced by smoking pure opium.

4.3 Europe: Alchemy and Science

Paracelsus (Theophrastus von Hohenheim, c1493-1541) was a Swiss physician and alchemist credited who was the 'father of toxicology'.

He is also credited with reintroducing opium to Western Europe in the form of a pill that he called 'Laudanum' (from the Latin meaning 'worthy of praise').

His Laudanum pills were also called 'stones of immortality' and described as a general purpose painkiller. The ingredients are listed as opium thebaicum, citrus juice, and quintessence of gold.

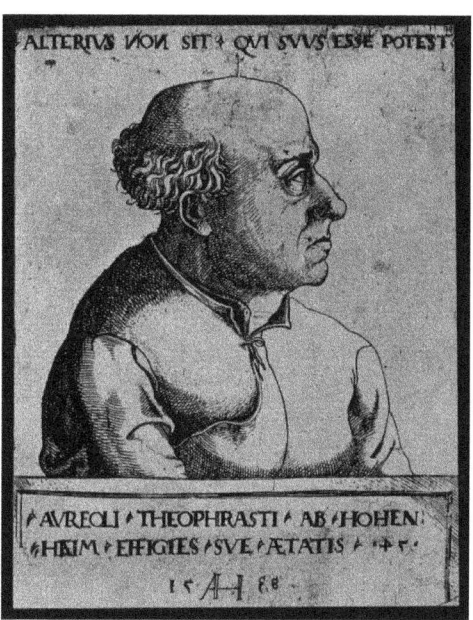

A portrait of Paracelsus by Augustin Hirschvogel, 1538

Thomas Sydenham (1624-1689) was an English physician who is referred to the 'father of English medicine'. He popularised a tincture of opium that he also named Laudanum, and encouraged its use for a range of medical conditions, including pain medication and as a cough suppressant, and to treat diarrhoea. It was also widely prescribed to women with menstrual cramps.

Several decades later, the medicinal properties of opium and laudanum were well known, and the term Laudanum came to mean any combination of opium and alchohol. Laudanum was sold without prescription up until the early 20th century in a variety of patented medicines.

As the population of cities in Europe continued to grow and expand, struggling with outdated and inadequate sanitation, outbreaks of cholera and dysentery were major threats to public health, with victims often dying from severe diarrhoea, dropsy (edema), consumption (tuberculosis), fever, and rheumatism.

Laudanum would have been very popular as it was cheaper than a bottle of gin, and though it contained alcohol, it was treated as a medication and not taxed as an alcoholic beverage.

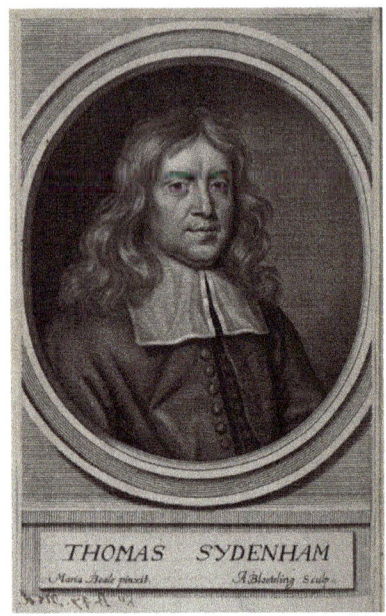

A Portrait of Thomas Sydenham Abraham Blooteling

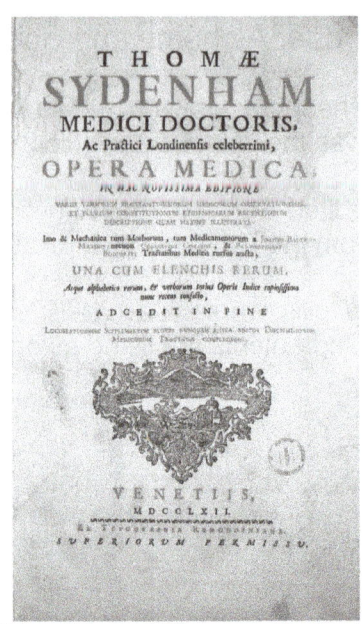

A 1762 edition of Thomas Sydenham's 'Opera Medica'

Ephraim Chambers (c1680-1740) was an English writer and encyclopaedist who in 1728 published the 'Cyclopædia, or an Universal Dictionary of Arts and Sciences'.

Use of opium as a cure-all was reflected in the formulation of mithridatium, a semi-mythical remedy with as many as 65 ingredients, used as an antidote to poison, said to be created by Mithridates VI Eupator of Pontus in the 1st century BCE. Among the many ingredients was opium.

From then on laudanum became the basis of many popular medicines of the 19th century.

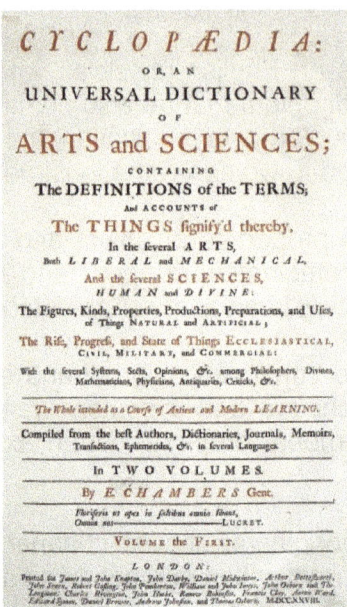

Ephraim Chambers's 'Cyclopaedia', 1728

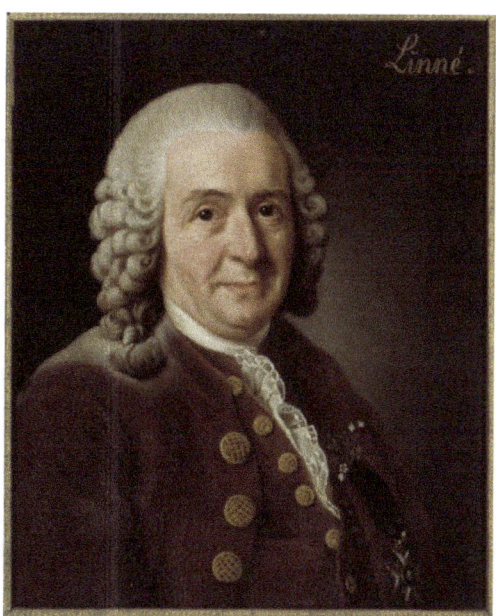

A portrait of Carl Linnaeus by Alexander Roslin, 1775

Carl Linnaeus (1701-1778) was a Swedish botanist and physician who is referred to as 'the father of botany'. In his books '*Species Plantarum*' and '*Genera Plantarum*', the opium poppy was first classified as '*Papaver Somniferum*'. Papaver is the Latin word for poppy, and somniferum means 'sleep inducing'.

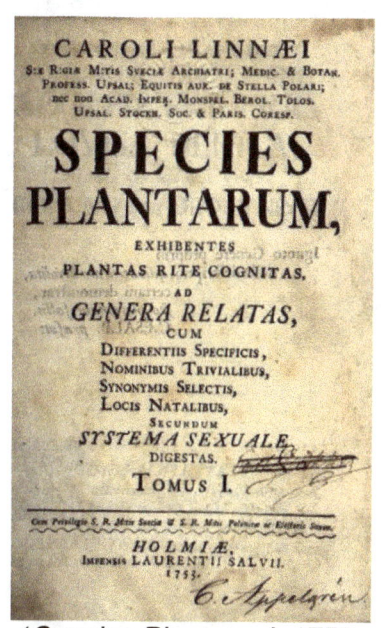

'*Species Plantarum*', 1753

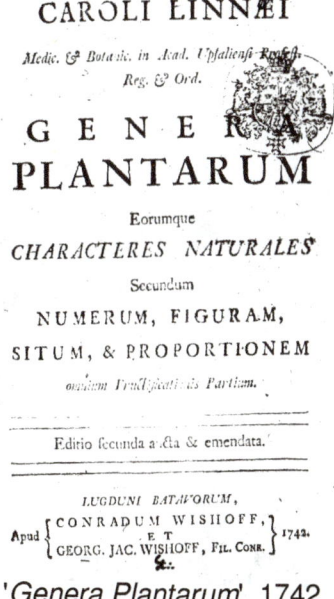

'*Genera Plantarum*', 1742

The classification *Papaver Somniferum* appeared in botanical publications from then on.

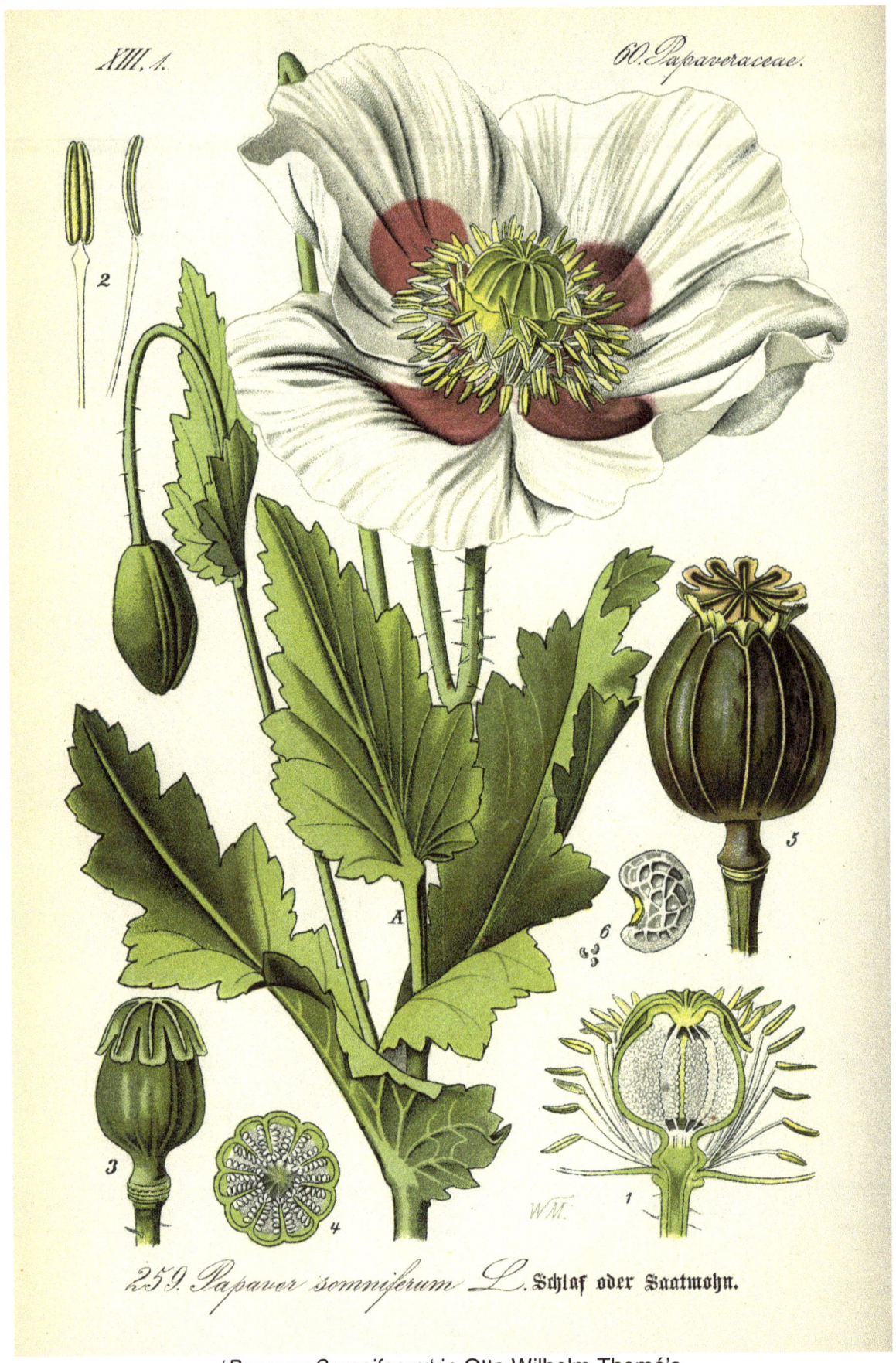

'*Papaver Somniferum*' in Otto Wilhelm Thomé's
'*Flora von Deutschland, Österreich und der Schweiz*', 1885

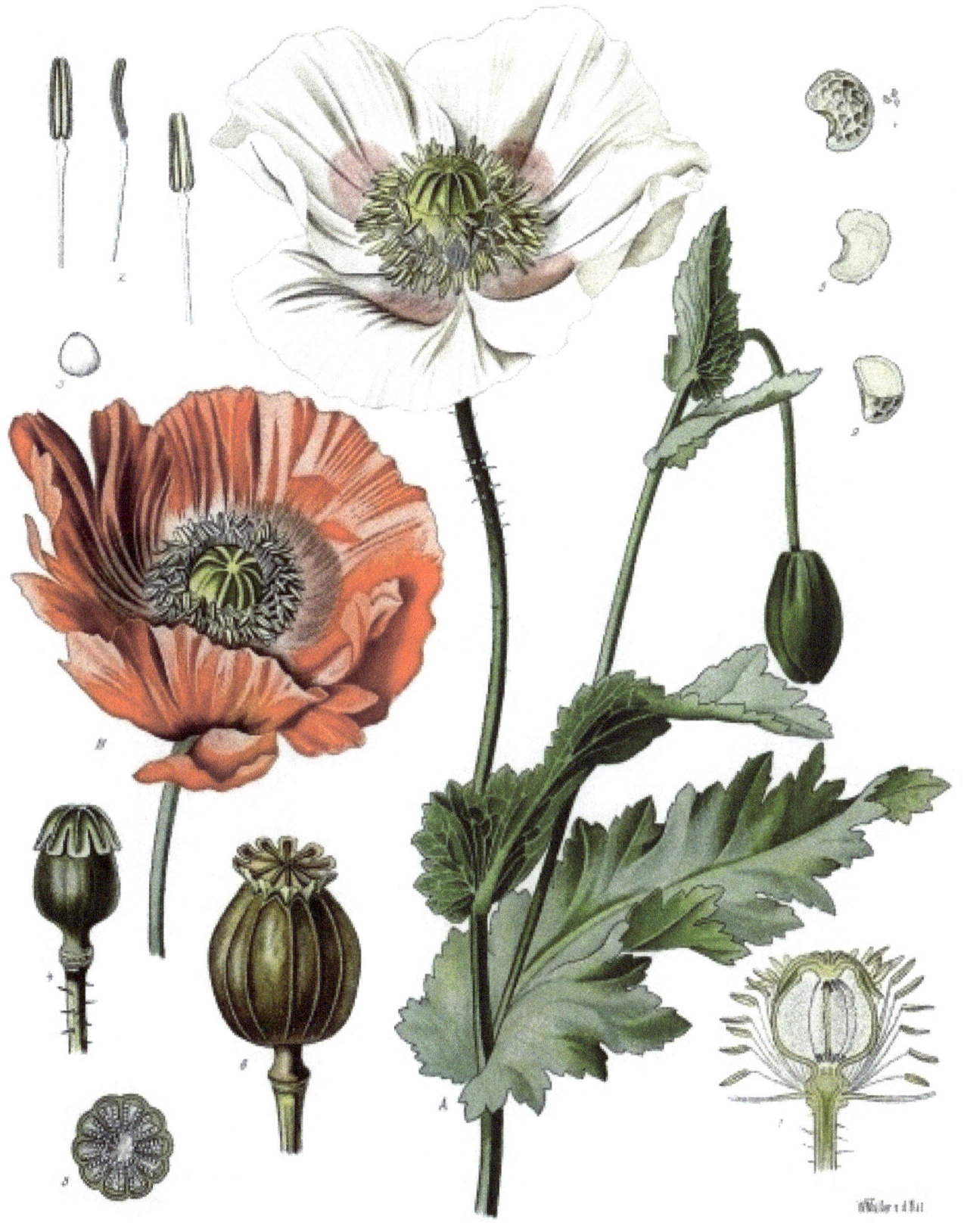

'*Papaver Somniferum*' in Franz Eugen Köhler's '*Köhler's Medizinal-Pflanzen*', 1897

4.4 New Trade Routes to the East

In the early 1400s Portugal was centre of exploration, navigation, and maritime expansion. It became necessary to look for new trade routes to the east, to avoid the stranglehold that the Venetians and the Ottomans had on the taxation of goods travelling East and West.

It was also hoped that expeditions would locate the legendary 'Spice Islands' in the East Indies and that Portuguese traders would be able to gain a foothold in the lucrative spice trade.

Henry the Navigator became known as the 'patron of Portuguese exploration'. With the latest cartography, instruments, and the latest ship the Caravel, voyages and expeditions explored further and further down the West African coast until Bartolomeu Dias reached the Cape of Good Hope, the southern tip of Africa in 1488.

In 1498 Vasco Da Gama became the first European to reach India by sea, arriving at Calicut on the Malabar coast of South West India. Footholds, factories, trading posts, and forts would appear across India, Southeast Asia, and China.

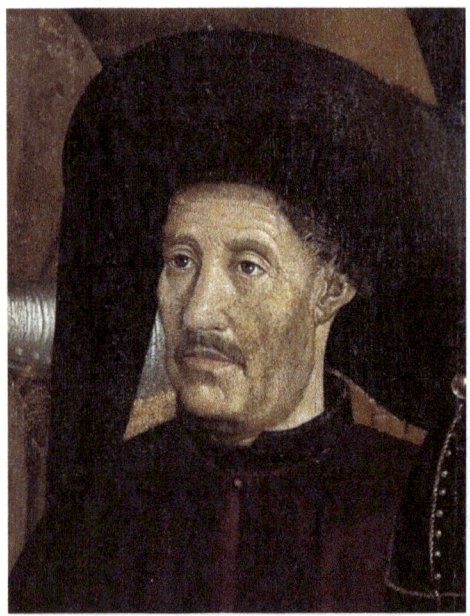

Henry the Navigator, detail from Saint Vincent Panels by Nuno Gonçalves, 15th Century

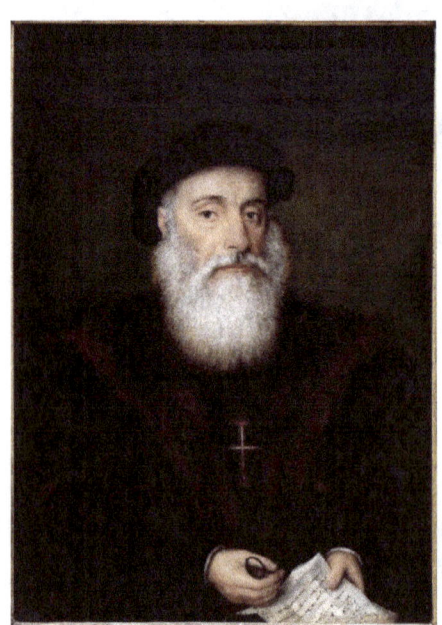

A 16th Century portrait of Vasco Da Gama

Afonso de Albuquerque conquered the Malaysian city of Malacca in 1511, which guaranteed access to the Malacca Strait, a narrow channel that connects The Indian Ocean to the South China Sea.

Jorge Álvares was the first European to reach China by sea in 1513, and Portugal extablished trading activities in southern China, which gradually expanded to Macau (Àomén), and then up the Pearl River to Canton (Guǎngzhōu). Rent or tribute was paid to the Ming Emperor Zhengde.

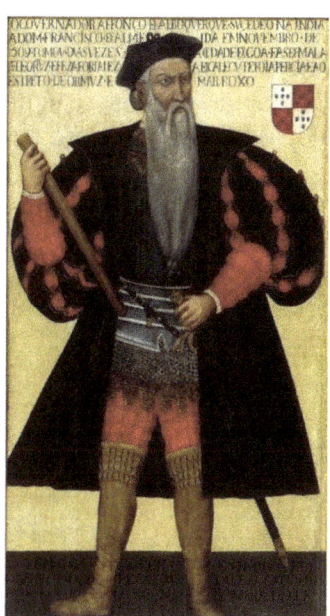

A Portait of Afonso de Albuquerque, after 1545

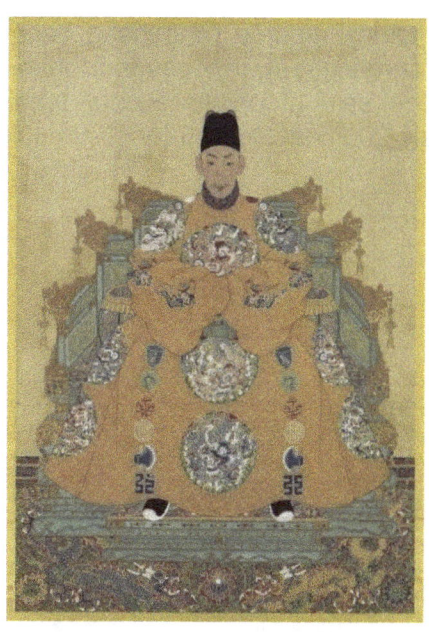

Ming Emperor Zhengde

As well as selling spices obtained from posts in Southeast Asia, merchants were able to transport Indian opium from their trading posts at Calicut, Goa, Chittagong, and Bombay to Macau, selling it to Chinese merchants.

The British East India Company was founded in the last days of the year 1600 to trade in the East Indies (The Indian Subcontinent and Southeast Asia) and later with Qing China. They established footholds in Banten (Java) and the Maluku Islands, also known as the 'Spice Islands'. The Dutch East India Company was formed soon after in 1602 to trade with Mughal India and Southeast Asian countries in the spice trade. By 1605 they had several footholds in India and Southeast Asia. The British and the Dutch began to compete aggressively with the Portuguese and with each other.

The practise of smoking opium was probably introduced to China by the Dutch, selling opium from Java, which was then blended with herbs, boiled, and then mixed with tobacco. The mixture was called 'Madak', and the practice caught on first in coastal areas in the Taiwain Strait, and then spread along the coast of Southern China.

The Ming Dynasty was replaced by the Qing Dynasty in 1644, and a series of rebellions were put down before the Qing Emperor Kangxi gave the following edict in 1684:

> "Now the whole country is unified, everywhere there is peace and quiet, Manchu-Han relations are fully integrated so I command you to go abroad and trade to show the populous and affluent nature of our rule. By imperial decree I open the seas to trade".

Formal permission was given for all Westerners to trade in in Chinese ports in 1685, and the Qing court set up a trading company to deal with Western trade known as the *Yánghuò Háng* (Ocean Trading House).

In 1704, the *Baoshang* system meant that Chinese merchants would visit to pay taxes due, and duties which they had collected from the Western merchants. Most Westerners chose to trade at Canton as it is closer to Southeast Asia and it was less profitable to travel further north. In 1715 the British East India Company factory was established at Canton.

In 1729 the Qing Emperor Yongzheng became disturbed by the amount of madak being smoked at court, and carrying out the government's role of upholding Confucian virtues, issued an edict prohibiting the sale of opium except small amounts for medicinal purposes, limiting imports to approximately 200 chests (12.5 tons) annually. Smoking pure opium became more popular from then on.

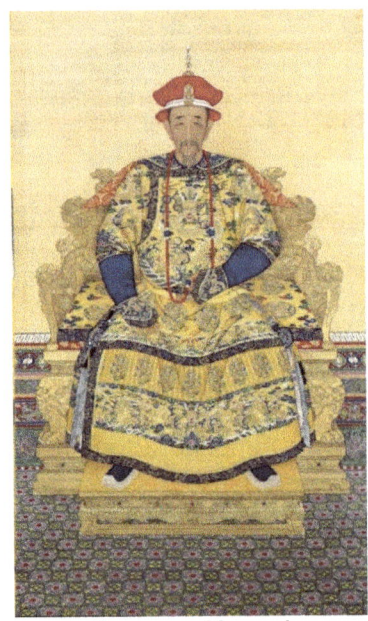

Emperor Kangxi

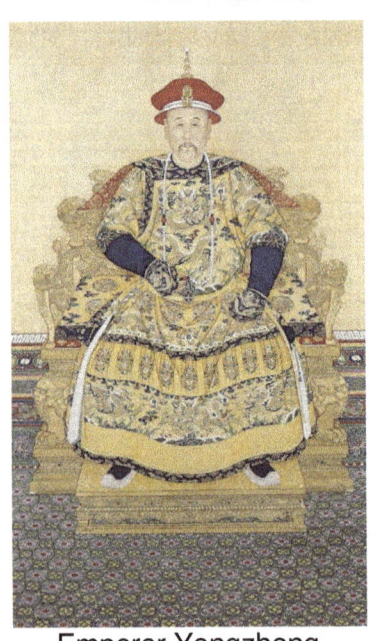

Emperor Yongzheng

Changes were implemented by the Qing Emperor Qianlong into what was called the Cohong system, where the Chinese merchant stood as guarantor for every foreign trading vessel entering Canton Harbour and any taxes due from the Western merchants.

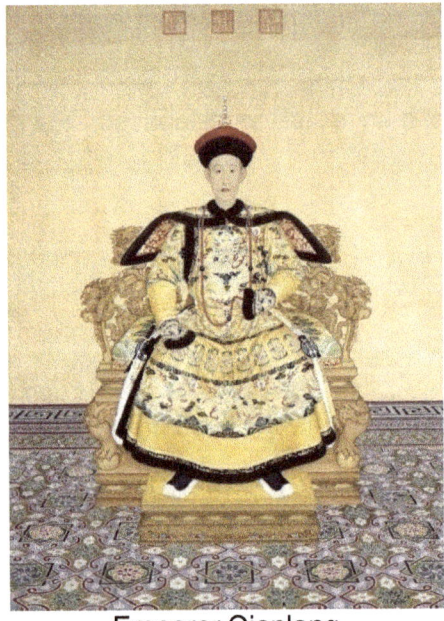

Emperor Qianlong

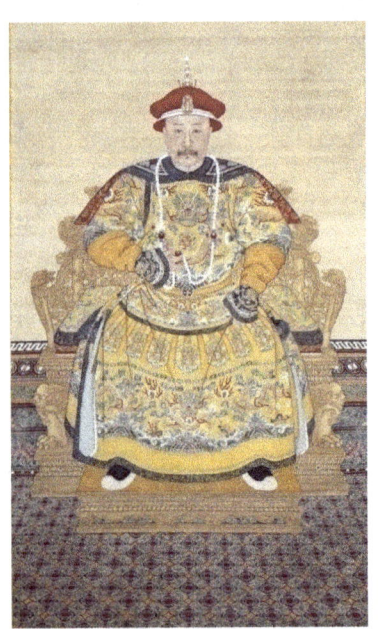

Emperor Jiaqing

Between 1750 and 1757, the British East India Company took control of Bengal and Bihar, two opium-growing districts of India. Shortly afterwards British shipping dominated the trade from Calcutta to

China, and a monopoly on that trade soon followed. Within 10 years, the British East India Company's import of Opium into China reached a staggering two thousand chests (124 tons) of opium per year.

An edict was issued in 1796 by Emperor Jiaqing prohibiting opium smoking, which was followed in 1799 by an edict banning opium altogether, making trade and poppy cultivation illegal.

In 1736 Huang Shujing was sent by Emperor Kangxi to Taiwan as the first Imperial High Commissioner. He recorded his findings in *Táihǎi shǐ chá lù* (Records from the mission to Taiwan and its Strait).

The smoking of pure opium was described as involving a pipe made from bamboo rimmed with silver, stuffed with palm slices and hair, fed by a clay bowl in which a globule of molten opium was held over the flame of an oil lamp.

This elaborate procedure, requiring the maintenance of pots of opium at just the right temperature for a globule to be scooped up with a needle-like skewer for smoking, formed the basis of a craft of "paste-scooping" which servants and prostitutes became proficient in as the opportunity arose.

4.5 Opium and Romanticism, Part 1

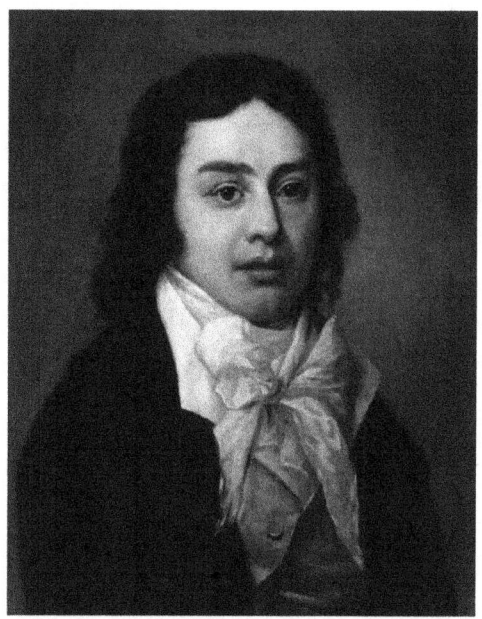

Samuel Taylor Coleridge by Peter Vandyke, 1795

Samuel Taylor Coleridge (1772-1834) was an English poet who was one of the founders of the Romantic Movement in England, along with his friend and fellow poet William Wordsworth.

The Romantic Movement is characterised by art, music, and literature that seeks to connect most immediately and most powerfully with the deepest of emotions, to speak directly to the soul, celebrating individualism, revisiting and glorifying by imagination scenes from the past, particularly in mythology, and being in harmony with nature.

Coleridge suffered with rheumatic fever, and crippling bouts of anxiety and depression. He was treated with laudanum, which resulted in his developing a lifelong addiction. In later years he was taking almost 300ml of laudanum a week.

In 1797 he wrote the poem 'Kubla Khan' one night after he experienced an opium-influenced dream after reading a work describing Shangdu, the summer capital of the Yuan Dynasty founded by the Mongol Emperor Kublai Khan. It was not published until 1816 at the insistence of his friend Lord Byron. The poem is well known for its vivid imagery, celebration of creativity, and as a poet, Coleridge wonders whether he is a master of his creative powers or a slave to them.

Kubla Khan Manuscript, 1797

*"And all who heard should see them there,
And all should cry, beware! Beware!
His flashing eyes, his floating hair!
Weave a circle around him thrice
And close four eyes with holy dread,
For he on honey-dew hath fed,
And drunk the milk of Paradise".*

Lines 48-54 of Coleridge's *'Kubla Khan'*

Coleridge's increasing dependence on laudanum plagued his personal life. He suffered frequent nightmares which robbed him of sleep. Marital problems and tensions with Wordsworth eventually alienated him from his family and friends.

He wrote in his poem '*Dejection: An Ode*' about having lost his ability to write poetry, and living in a state of paralysis, unable to enjoy nature.

> "*My genial spirits fail;*
>   *And what can these avail*
> *To lift the smothering weight from off my breast?*
>   *It were a vain endeavour,*
>   *Though I should gaze for ever*
> *On that green light that lingers in the west:*
> *I may not hope from outward forms to win*
> *The passion and the life, whose fountains are within*".

Part 3, lines 39-46 of Coleridge's 'Dejection: An Ode'

The Romantic Era was a time of growth for the arts and for opium use. The reported euphoric psychological effects that accompanied the use of opiates meant that more and more people were using it recreationally as well as for medicinal purposes.

The day-dream like trance was thought to open a channel of creativity in the mind between the conscious and the subconscious, and allow greater access to visions of the imagination which could be used for creative and artistic purposes.

For some, opium was part of the fascination in all things from the East, which was still characterised in the imagination as an exotic place of mystery, extravagance, opulence, and decadence.

This was partly because of the wealth of travel literature that had been popular since the Middle Ages, including such tales of the orient, accounts of journeys to foreign lands in the east, with vivid descriptions of architecture, art, kings and queens, costume and customs, which most readers could only dream of seeing for themselves.

The opiates that were believed to inspire creativity of the mind ultimately became the poison that extinguished and destroyed it.

5. The 19th Century Part 1: *Culture, Science, and Art (1800-1839)*

5.1 Opium in the East: The Smoking Ritual

In China and Southeast Asia the tradition of opium smoking continued to flourish, and was seen as a very civilised pastime, primarily enjoyed by the wealthy scholars, bureaucrats, and gentry, then gradually moving down the social classes to landowners, merchants, artisans, workers and peasants.

The sophisticated tastes of the wealthy led to ever more elaborate paraphernalia being used, with more and more exotic and expensive materials, employing increasingly intricate detail and artistic skill in their design. Such accoutrements became a way of demonstrating a person's wealth and standing in society. Opium was offered as a form of greeting and politeness, and often served with tea in China.

The Opium Pipe has two parts, first of all is the smoking tube, one end of which is sealed with a plug usually made of ivory, jade, bone, or marble, and the other end has a fitted mouthpiece usually made of the same material. The second part is the damper bowl or 'head', usually round and made of terracotta or porcelain, also found in a variety of other shapes and with ever varied decoration. The job of the damper is to act as a chamber that allows the smoke to cool before it reaches the mouthpiece. At the bottom of the bowl is a small stem, which is designed to fit snugly inside a metal collar or 'saddle' usually in copper, bronze, silver, or an intricate combination.

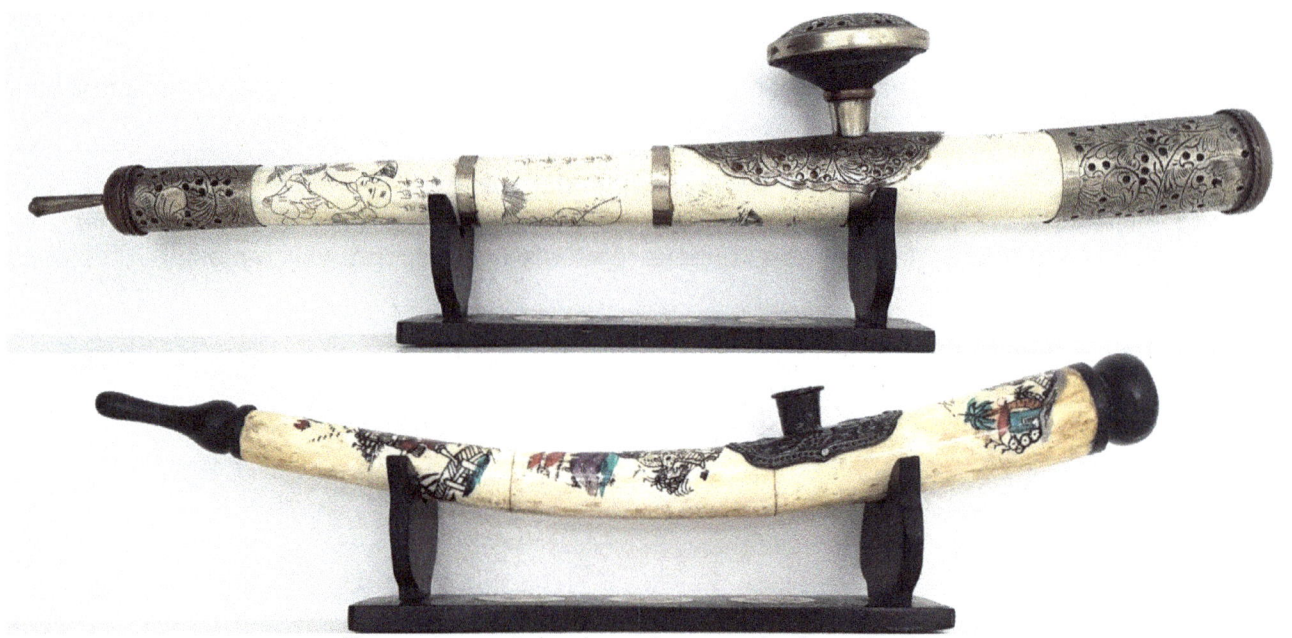

Two ornamental opium pipes, author's collection

The Opium Lamp is made up of a metal stand with an oil chamber at the bottom, made of copper, brass, or porcelain. A wick is held in place at the top of the oil chamber in a small collar that fits in place over the rim at the opening, where the wick suspends down into the chamber and conducts the oil upwards to feed the flame, which must be as small as possible to provide a slow steady low heat with as little smoke as possible. A glass chimney sits on the top of the stand and channels the rising heat of the flame into a small narrow opening where the heat is concentrated. The glass at the top of the chimney thickens considerably, both to narrow the channel to and reinforce the glass. This is the main difference between the opium lamp and traditional oil lamps of the same period.

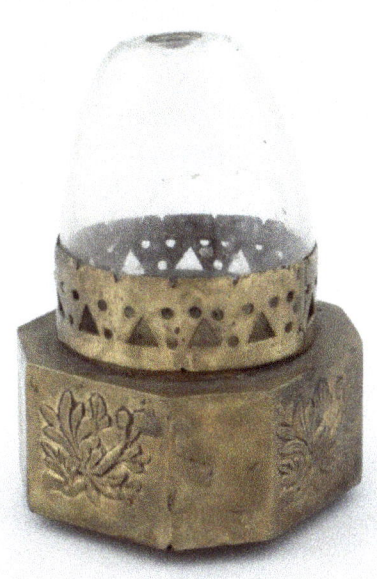 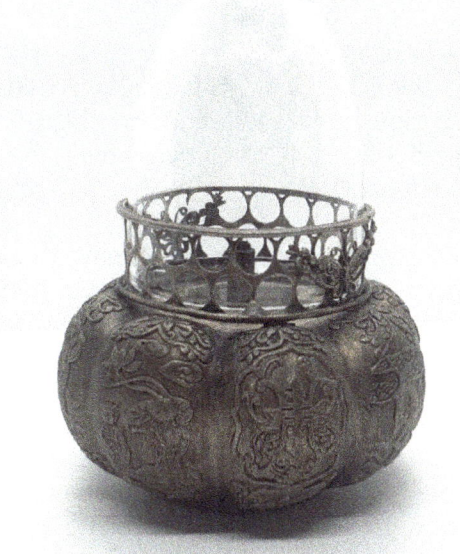

A typical brass opium lamp | A traditional Chinese oil lamp, author's collection

The metal stand must allow a small amount of air into the chimney at the base to travel upwards with the flame, or there will not be enough oxygen to sustain the flame. The wick must also be trimmed regularly to ensure a steady flame while burning.

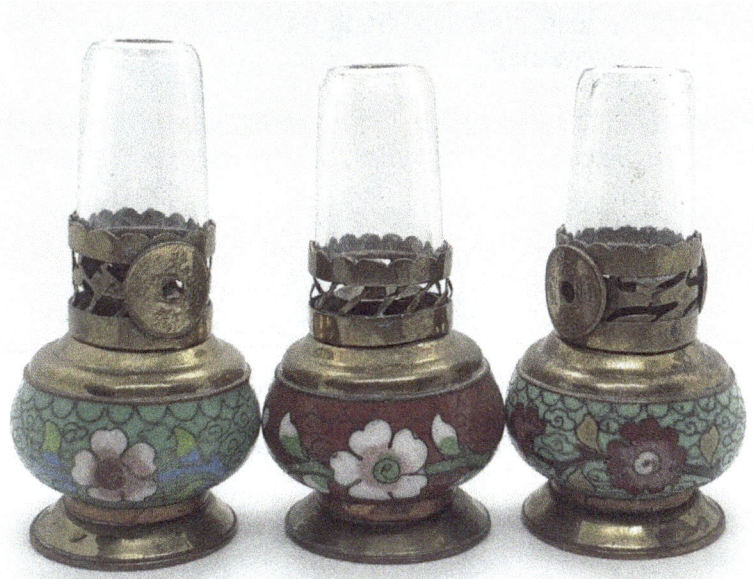

Three vintage small opium lamps in brass with enamel cloisonné decoration, author's collection

When the opium is shaped into a small pellet and placed on the damper bowl of the pipe, a skewer or spindle is used to pierce a hole through the pellet into the bowl. The bowl of the pipe is then placed over the lamp to gently heat the opium. The hole in the opium pellet allows the emanating vapours to be drawn into the pipe and then inhaled. Afterwards the leftover opium called 'dross' is cleaned from the bowl using scraping tools. Poorer opium smokers at the bottom end of the social classes who could not afford opium had the opportunity to smoke the collected and reshaped dross which was of lower quality.

5.2 Opium in the West: Science and Addiction

Friedrich Wilhelm Adam Sertürner (1783-1841) was a German pharmacist and a pioneer of alkaloid chemistry. Alkaloids are the active ingredients in plants used for medicine that can influence circulation, digestion, respiration, and also act directly on tissue and organs of the human body with physiological effects. Some can affect the central nervous system producing psychological and emotional effects.

In previous centuries, plants containing these alkaloids were known to shamans and alchemists as 'power plants'. The bio-active substances had no other use in the lives of the plants in which they were found, and they were specially designed to mirror that which regulates the human body and affect its functions. These gifts of nature were part of the important relationship between the divine, humankind, and nature.

In Paderborn, Germany in December 1804 Sertürner began investigating the possibility of isolating the alkaloids of opium. The successful process involved dissolving the opium in acid, and then neutralising it with ammonia. He called the resulting salt-like substance 'morphium' after the ancient Greek word μορφή 'morphḗ' (form or shape) from which the name of the Greek and Roman god Morpheus 'the shaper of dreams' is related.

The possibility of isolating these alkaloids led to the belief that opium had finally perfected and tamed. Now that it had been isolated, the exact dose could be controlled, rather than being dependant on the variable amount of morphine contained in the latex of each poppy.

Morphium was six times stronger than opium, and Sertürner believed that, because lower doses of the drug were needed, it would be less addictive. Sadly however, this was not the case, and as he became addicted to morphine. He warned:

"I consider it my duty to attract attention to the terrible effects of this new substance I called morphium in order that calamity may be averted".

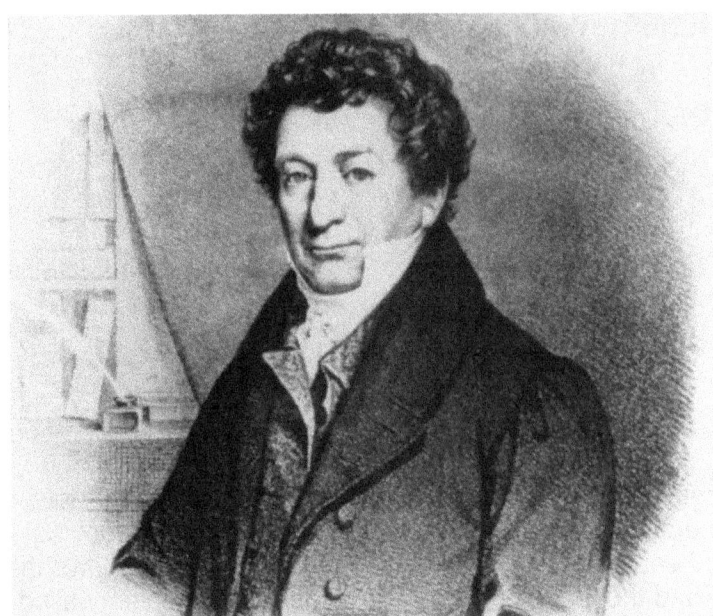

A lithograph of Friedrich Wilhelm Adam Sertürner, c1830-1840

The six main alkaloids isolated from opium used in medicine are morphine, codeine, thebaine, papaverine, narcotine, and narceine. The amount of each of these alkaloids in opium can vary as much as follows (approximate):

Alkaloid	Low	High	Description
Morphine	3.0%	24.0%	Morphine acts directly on the central nervous system, fitting into the endorphin receptors in the brain and anesthetising channels in the spinal cord and brain stem. It slows respiration, relaxes the bronchial system, suppresses appetite and impedes digestive functions, decreases body temperature, and inhibits perspiration.
Codeine	0.4%	1.0%	Codeine has painkilling properties but less than morphine. It causes restful sleep which makes it a popular remedy for acute respiratory ailments in which painful and uncontrollable coughing and chronic lung congestion keep the patient awake at night.
Thebaine	0.4%	0.8%	Thebaine acts as a cerebral stimulant and counteracts the sleep-inducing effects of morphine and codeine.
Papaverine	0.4%	0.8%	Papaverine acts as a relaxant to the involuntary muscles of the body, and particularly the muscles that control the walls of blood vessels, so much so that it significantly increases blood flow throughout the circulatory system right down to the smallest capillaries.
Narcotine	4.0%	7.0%	Narcotine functions as a stimulant and accelerates respiration, counteracting the respiratory suppressant effects of morphine.
Narceine	0.2%	0.5%	Narceine has mild sleep-inducing effects similar to morphine and codeine, but less strong.

In 1827, E Merck & Company of Darmstadt, Germany, began commercial manufacturing of morphine which soon became very popular as a pain killer and a cough decongestant.

5.3 Opium and Romanticism, Part 2

In the novel Frankenstein written by Mary Shelley (1797-1851) the character Victor Frankenstein describes his use of laudanum:

> *"Ever since my recovery from the fever, I had been in the custom of taking every night a small quantity of laudanum, for it was by means of this drug only that I was enabled to gain the rest necessary for the preservation of life. Oppressed by the recollection of my various misfortunes, I now swallowed double my usual quantity and soon slept profoundly. But sleep did not afford me respite from thought and misery; my dreams presented a thousand objects that scared me. Towards morning I was possessed by a kind of nightmare;"*

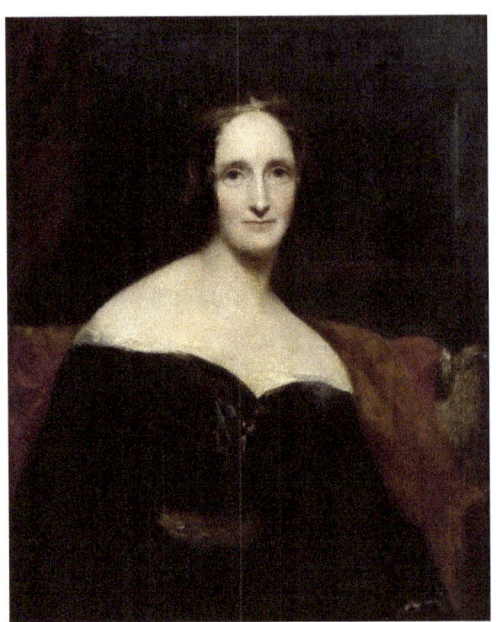

Mary Shelley by Richard Rothwell, c1840

Romantic poet John Keats (1795-1821) wrote one of the most famous and beautifully moving poems '*Ode to a Nightingale*' in 1819, which was published in 1820. Critics have interpreted it as a reference to Keats's experience with laudanum.

> *"My heart aches, and a drowsy numbness pains*
> *My sense, as though of hemlock I had drunk,*
> *Or emptied some dull opiate to the drains*
> *One minute past, and Lethe-wards had sunk:"*

The drowsy numbness is the effect of the laudanum. The hemlock is a reference to ancient Greece, where hemlock was a poison given to condemned prisoners, or mixed with raw opium and used to commit suicide.

The dull opiate is laudanum, and '*Lethe*' in this case refers in Greek mythology to the river of forgetfulness in the underworld.

As he begins to fall into a trance, he hears a bird singing in the distance, and so he yearns for poetic inspiration to help him to escape the "the weariness the fever, and the fret" of the present, and like the bird "with thee fade away into the forest dim".

He muses on where this flight of poetic fancy will take him, and begins to describe the imagined landscape around him, despite the fact that his "dull brain perplexes and retards".

His use of the word "forlorn" reminds him of his own sadness, and he is immediately pulled back to the present moment, as the birdsong fades into the distance, and he is left wondering "do I wake or sleep?"

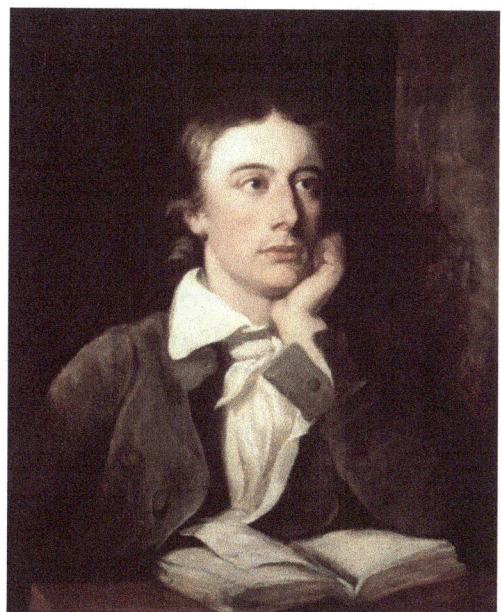

John Keats by William Hilton, c1822

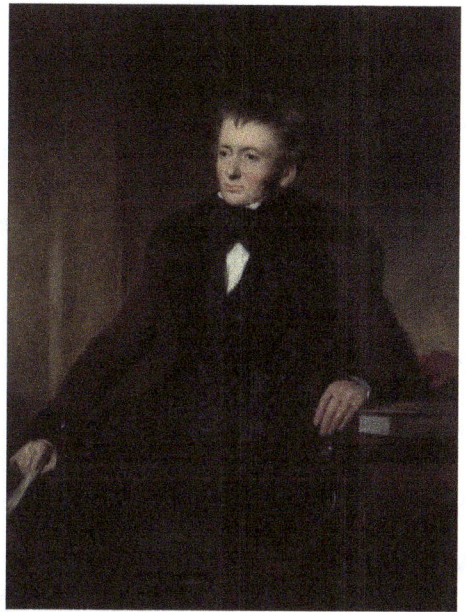

Thomas De Quincey by John Watson Gordon, c1846

Thomas De Quincey published his autobiographical account of opium addiction in 'Confessions of an English Opium-Eater' in 1821, which started with the relief of a toothache in 1804.

He is initially full of praise and wonder at its effectiveness, but later as his story unfolds he becomes philosophical of the danger of its addiction.

> *"Thou hast the keys of Paradise, O just, subtle, and mighty opium!"*

> *"Nobody will laugh long who deals much with opium: its pleasures even are of a grave and solemn complexion".*

6. The Opium Wars: *East and West Collide (1839-1860)*

6.1 Diplomacy and Trade

Since the early 17th century the British had gradually developed a massive appetite for tea. It was first noted as an exotic curiosity, then gained popularity as a luxury drink among the upper-classes with medicinal properties, and gradually spread through all social classes to become vitally important part of British culture and national identity. Tea was only available from China, and all the trade was channelled through the Canton System. The British East India Company had a monopoly on Britain's tea trade with China, and the tea could only be purchased with silver. As Britain's supplies of silver decreased, this presented a problem for the British economy.

British merchants lobbied the government to send an embassy to China to secure favourable changes to existing arrangements. A mission was arranged with the aim of persuading the Qianlong Emperor to open new ports for British trade in China, establish a permanent embassy in Peking (Běijīng), grant the use of a small island for the British along China's coast, and relax trade restrictions on British merchants in Canton. It was also hoped that a selection of gifts presented before the Qing court would showcase British advances in science and technology, and products which China might wish to accept in trade for tea instead of silver.

On the 14th September 1793 the Macartney Embassy met the Qianlong Emperor. Macartney refused to observe the ritual of the Kowtow (Kòutóu) which involved kneeling before the emperor and touching the head on the ground. Instead he bowed on one knee, as he would before his own king. In the end, due to cultural differences, a lack of knowledge, and disagreements regarding the status of both parties, the mission was unsuccessful. An edict from the Qianlong Emperor to King George III responded to the requests describing them as:

> "*contrary to all usage of my dynasty and cannot possibly be entertained*".

And regarding the gifts and products:

> "*Our Celestial Empire possesses all things in prolific abundance and lacks no product within its borders. There is therefore no need to import the manufactures of outside barbarians in exchange for our own produce*".

On the 29th August 1816 the Amherst Embassy was even less successful. He refused to perform the kowtow before the Emperor, unless it was formally acknowledged that his sovereign was entitled to the same show of reverence from a mandarin (bureaucrat or scholar) of the same rank as him. This was rejected, and he was refused entry into Beijing.

Despite the Chinese ban on opium, the demand continued, along with the lucrative trade to supply it. The British East India Company did not carry the opium itself, but instead licensed 'country traders' to transport the opium between India and China. The country traders sold the opium to smugglers along the Chinese coast in return for silver, which was then handed back to the British East India Company, who then used it to buy the tea, silk, and porcelain that could be sold profitably in back in the West in a form of 'triangular trade'. The amount of opium smuggled into China increased dramatically and the balance of trade shifted back in Britain's favour providing between 15% and 20% of the British Empire's revenues. China's supply of silver decreased, and the amount of opium addicts in China rose sharply, taking its toll on the fabric of Chinese society.

THE STACKING ROOM,
OPIUM FACTORY AT PATNA, INDIA.

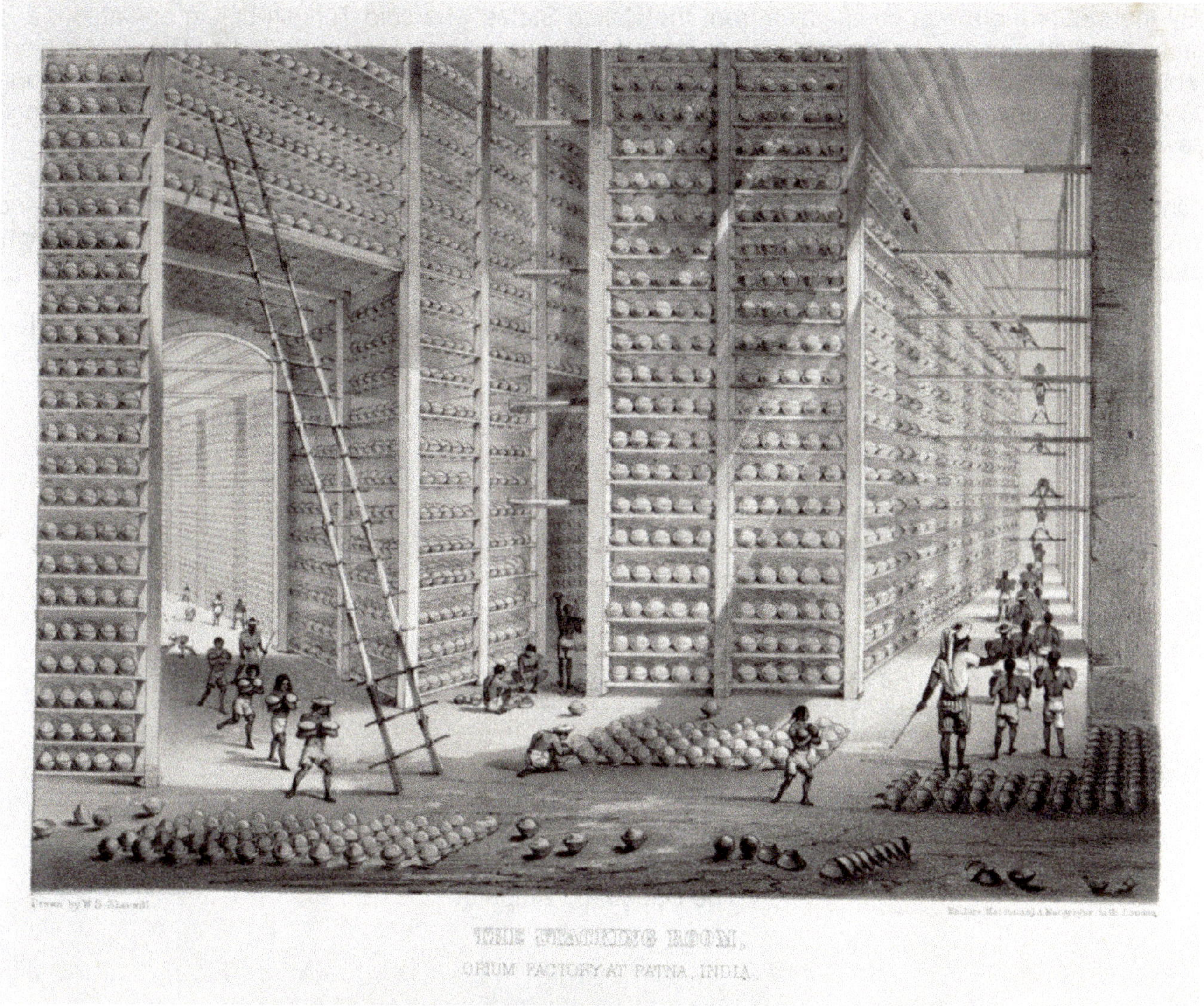

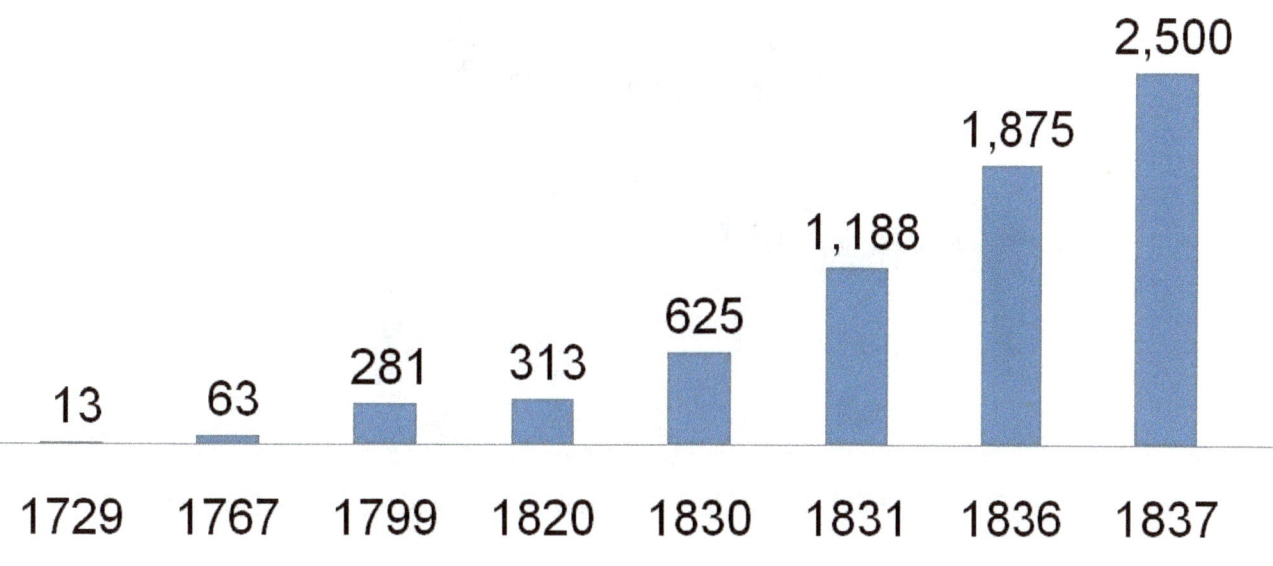

A stacking room at the opium factory in Patna, India, c1820

13
63
281
313
625
1,188
1,875
2,500
1729
1767
1799
1820
1830
1831
1836
1837

Opium imports into China by year in tons

By the 1820s there was competition from the United States who sold Turkish opium at Canton, and from the Portuguese who brought opium from the Malwa states of Western India. The British were able to restrict other trade by charging 'pass duty' on all vessels that were forced to pass through Bombay, which was under British rule. The British East India Company also increased production and lowered the price of opium in an attempt to edge out the competition.

On the 3rd October 1820 the Daoguang Emperor came to the throne and inherited the growing problem of the opium trade, rising addiction rates across the empire, and concerns of moral and social decay.

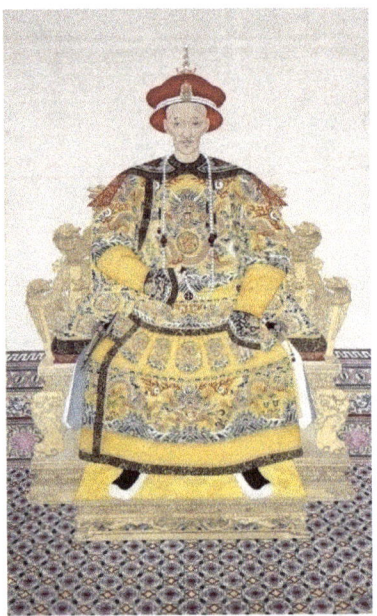

The Daoguang Emperor

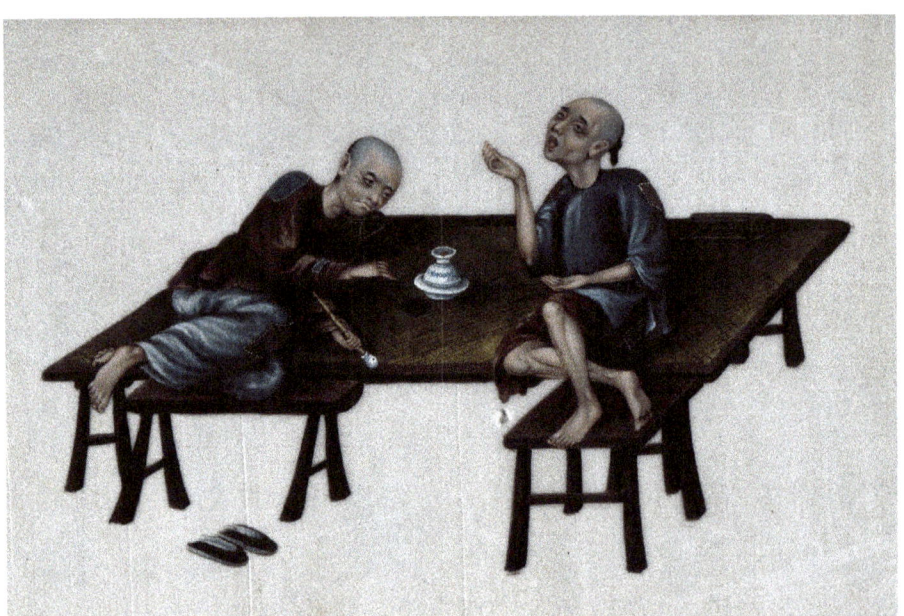

Two poor Chinese opium smokers, Gouache painting on rice-paper, 19th century.

In 1821 the tea trade was stopped for two months in an attempt to stop the opium trade. Opium dealers were punished with fines, imprisonment, and exile to the bleak landscape of Central Asia, ships were seized, cargo was confiscated and merchants were forbidden to trade in tea.

The Chinese authorities could make their presence felt on shore, but at sea they were powerless to stop the trade, and ways were found around new levels of enforcement.

Stocks of opium were regularly moved from one safe house to another, and chests were disguised as carrying other legal goods, and the small mountainous Lintin Island (*Nèi Língdīng Dǎo*) in Canton Bay was chosen as a depot for smugglers. Ships would discharge chests of opium and then carry on up the river with legal goods.

Lord Napier arrived in Macau in 1834 as the first Chief Superintendent of Trade at Canton, with the mission of expanding British trade into inner China. He lacked diplomatic and commercial experience, and failed to secure a meeting with Lu Kun, the Governor-general of the Lianguang (Liǎngguǎng).

He became frustrated at the trade deadlock and sent a dispatch to Foreign Secretary Lord Palmerston recommending a commercial treaty backed by an armed force. He recommended that the island of Hong Kong (Hēung Góng) should be taken as it is "admirably adapted for every purpose".

Napier sent *HMS Andromache* and *HMS Imogene* to Whampoa (Huángbù) on the 11th September 1834, defying an edict issued by Lu Kun, breaching defences at the Bocca Tigris (Hǔmén) on the Pearl River Delta (Zhūjiāng Sānjiǎozhōu). A skirmish of cannon fire led to a stalemate, and Lord Napier became ill with typhus and retired to Macau where he died of the fever on the 11th October 1834.

By this time, the British East India Company came under increasing criticism. Questions were asked about the legitimacy of its monopoly on trade. Since the battle of Plassey in 1757 and the territorial gains in India that followed, the company's activities had taken on an increasingly military and political role.

This was far away from the company's founding idea of 'trade not conquest'. Britain continued to support the company, sending troops when needed, particularly as the British conflict with France led to flashpoints around the world.

The Charter Act 1813 had renewed The British East India Company's charter, but ended its commercial monopoly, except for the tea and opium trade, and trade with China.

The Charter Act 1833 ended the activities of the company as a commercial body, and its monopoly on trade with China and other parts of the Far East, but it continued as an administrative body until it was formally dissolved on the 1st June 1874.

The vacuum left by the departure of the British East India Company was filled by Jardine, Matheson & Co. which quickly became the largest British trading firm in Asia, trading cotton, tea, silk, and opium.

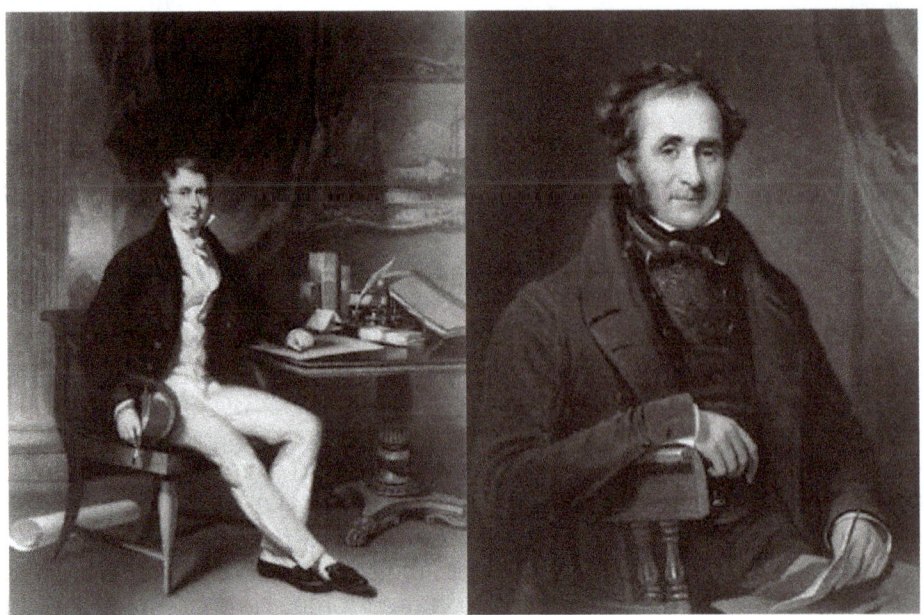

William Jardine and James Matheson

6.2 The Crackdown on Opium

Between 1836 and 1838 the amount of opium imported into China went from approximately 30,000 chests (1,875 tons) to approximately 40,000 chests (2,500 tons). The Qing court debate about the opium trade and legal measures against opium smugglers intensified, and proposals to legalise and tax opium were rejected.

Lin Zexu (*Lín Zéxú*) was a High-Commissioner of the Qing court who was tasked with ending the opium trade. He was praised for his strong moral conviction and incorruptibility, but was also criticised for his rigid approach, which did not take into account the international complexities of the problem. He wrote a letter to Queen Victoria appealing to her moral responsibility to stop the opium trade, but this letter never reached her.

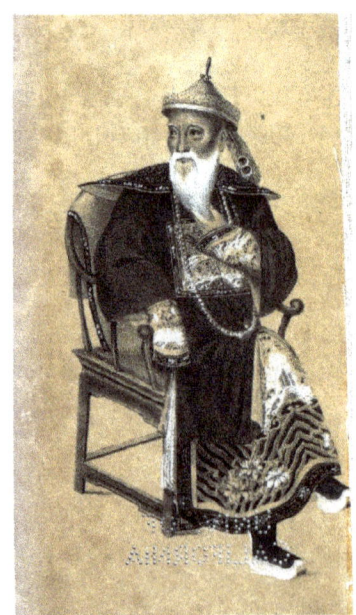

A portrait of Lin Zexu, c1843

"We find that your country is distant from us about sixty or seventy thousand miles, that your foreign ships come hither striving the one with the other for our trade, and for the simple reason of their strong desire to reap a profit. Now, out of the wealth of our Inner Land, if we take a part to bestow upon foreigners from afar, it follows, that the immense wealth which the said foreigners amass, ought properly speaking to be portion of our own native Chinese people.

By what principle of reason then, should these foreigners send in return a poisonous drug, which involves in destruction those very natives of China? Without meaning to say that the foreigners harbor such destructive intentions in their hearts, we yet positively assert that from their inordinate thirst after gain, they are perfectly careless about the injuries they inflict upon us! And such being the case, we should like to ask what has become of that conscience which heaven has implanted in the breasts of all men?"

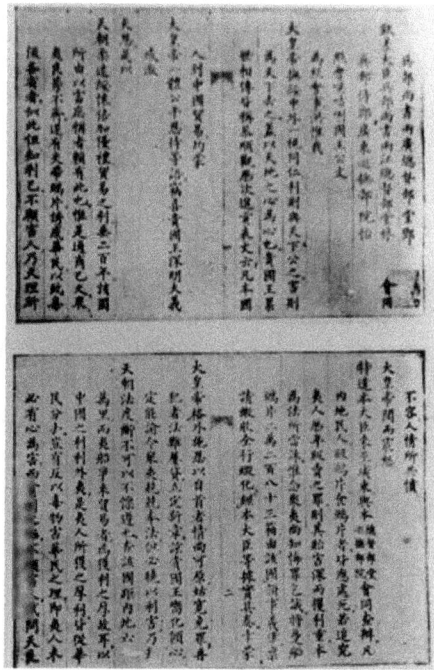

Lin Zexu's letter to Queen Victoria

On the 18th March 1839, the Daoguang Emperor issued the following edict:

"Any foreigner or foreigners bringing opium to the Central Land, with design to sell the same, the principals shall most assuredly be decapitated, and the accessories strangled; and all property (found on board the same ship) shall be confiscated.

The space of a year and a half is granted, within the which, if any one bringing opium by mistake, shall voluntarily step forward and deliver it up, he shall be absolved from all consequences of his crime".

When Lin arrived in Canton, the Pearl River was blockaded, Chinese troops boarded boats seizing and destroying opium, and merchants were trapped in their factories until they surrendered their opium stocks.

In order to end the blockade, Chief Superintendent Charles Elliot persuaded the merchants to hand over their opium, with the promise that the British government would compensate them for their loss.

The amount seized came to approximately 1,267 tons, which was publicly destroyed in front of Chinese court officials and foreign dignitaries. It took 500 workers 22 days to dispose of it all.

Elliot's promise of compensation for the merchants' losses had not been agreed by the British government, and it was thought that the Chinese government should pay the compensation.

In the frustration some merchants turned to William Jardine who believed that open warfare was the only way to obtain compensation from the Qing authorities, and he began campaigning to sway the British government.

In Canton, the sale of food to the British was banned. Chinese labourers in British Macau were withdrawn, war junks arrived along the Pearl River, and notices above the fresh water springs warned that they had been poisoned.

The Portuguese at Macau were ordered by the Chinese to expel the British from the colony, and the merchant fleet headed for Hong Kong.

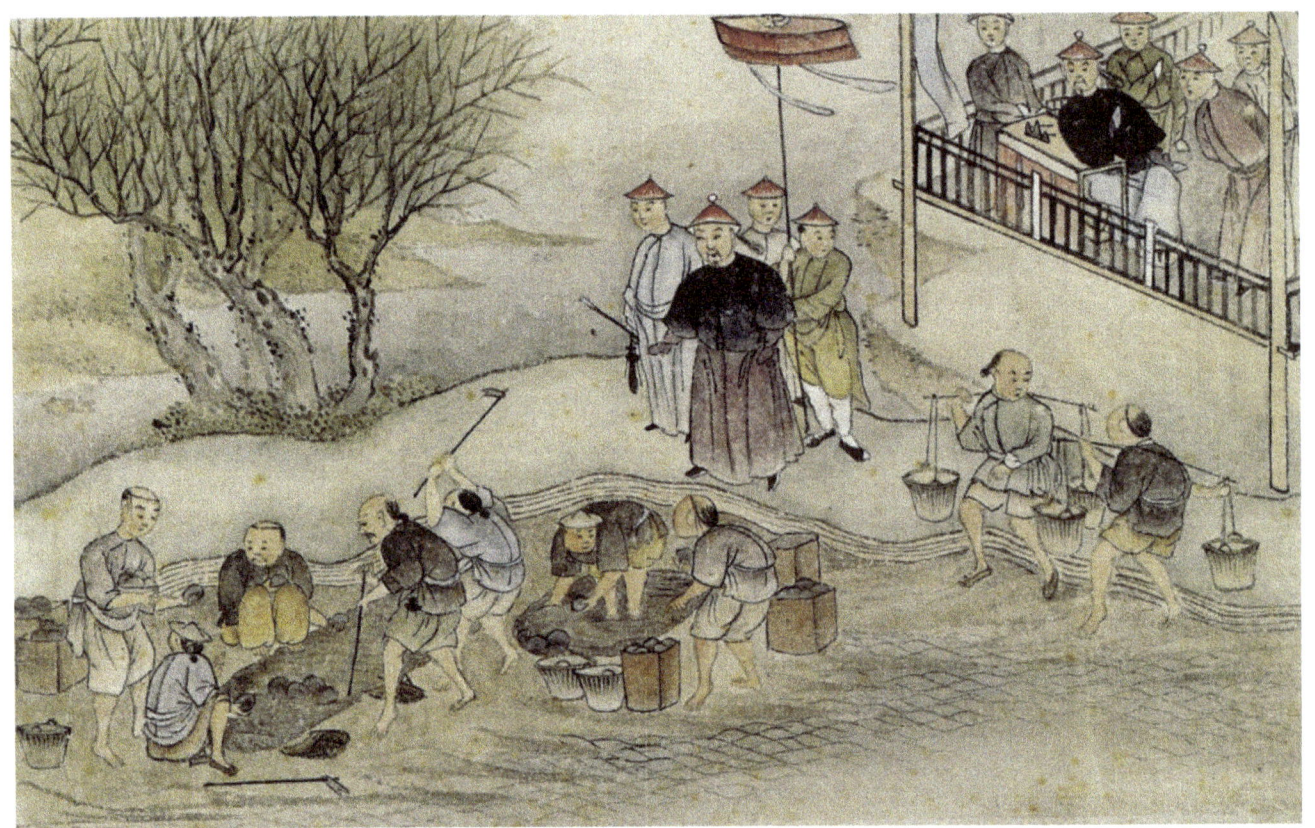

Commissioner Lin and the destruction of opium at Humen, June 1839

6.3 Voices of Opposition

British reaction to these events was mixed. Many British citizens were outraged that Britain was supporting the opium trade, and were sympathetic to the Chinese and thought that the sale of opium should be halted. There were also voices who spoke out against the notion of war with China, and against the trade between China and British India in general. Very few Tory or Liberal politicians supported the war. Sir James Graham, Lord Philip Stanhope, and William Ewart Gladstone were at the head of the anti-war faction in Britain.

Sir James Graham put forward a motion expressing severe disapproval of the Government's *"want of foresight"*, and *"their neglect to furnish the superintendent at Canton with powers and instructions"* to deal with the opium trade.

William Ewart Gladstone famously described the trade as *"most infamous and atrocious"*, and went on to say:

> *"A war more unjust in its origins, a war more calculated in its progress to cover this country with permanent disgrace, I do not know and have not read of".*

Charles Elliot himself was against the opium trade, but as someone who had already served for 24 years in the Royal Navy, he followed his orders to the letter. In one such letter to Foreign Secretary Lord Palmerston, he wrote:

> *"No man entertains a deeper detestation of the disgrace and sin of this forced traffic on the coast of China. I have steadily discountenanced it by all the lawful means in my power, and at the total sacrifice of my private comfort in the society in which I have lived for some years past".*

On the 8th April, after three days of debate, the pro-war lobby narrowly won by 271 votes to 262. The motion had failed by 9 votes to deter the Government from proceeding with the war and stopping the expeditionary force which was already on its way.

6.4 The First Opium War

China did not have a unified navy, but instead had a system of naval defences managed by each of the provinces, designed to counter the threat of pirates in close range river engagements. Gun forts looked imposing and impressive, but the large heavy guns were fixed and could not be aimed, and with less range they were of little use against a highly mobile and manoeuvrable force.

The British warships carried more guns and they were more manoeuvrable, and British tactics had been honed in the Napoleonic Wars and the colonial wars of the 1820s and 1830s. Many of the soldiers were veterans of colonial wars in India and had experience of fighting larger armies.

The British formula for gunpowder was of better quality with more sulphur giving them a greater range which allowed them the space to attack the Chinese forts with little risk to themselves. Faced with superior firepower, the Chinese were only able to offer limited resistance before sailing away or abandoning their posts, as detachments of marines and sailors landed and captured forts and guns.

The British made their way up the East coast of China, finally capturing Chinkiang (Zhènjiāng) on the 21st July 1842. This had strategic importance as it allowed the British to block the intersection of the Yangtze River (Cháng Jiāng) and the Jing–Hang Grand Canal (Jīng-Háng Dà Yùnhé), disrupting movement of grain throughout the empire, and offering a canal route to Peking. British forces then gathered at Nanking (Nánjīng).

The Daoguang Emperor was forced to sue for peace, and after two weeks, the Treaty of Nanking (Nánjīng Tiáoyuē) was signed on the 29th August 1842 aboard the *HMS Cornwallis*. Hong Kong was ceded to the British, and five treaty ports were established for foreign trade: Amoy (Xiàmén), Canton, Fuchow (Fúzhōu), Ningpo (Níngbō), and Shanghai (Shànghǎi).

This was followed on the 8th October 1843 by the The Treaty of the Bogue, which was signed on the 8th October 1843 and granted extraterritoriality to Britain, and the status of most favoured nation.

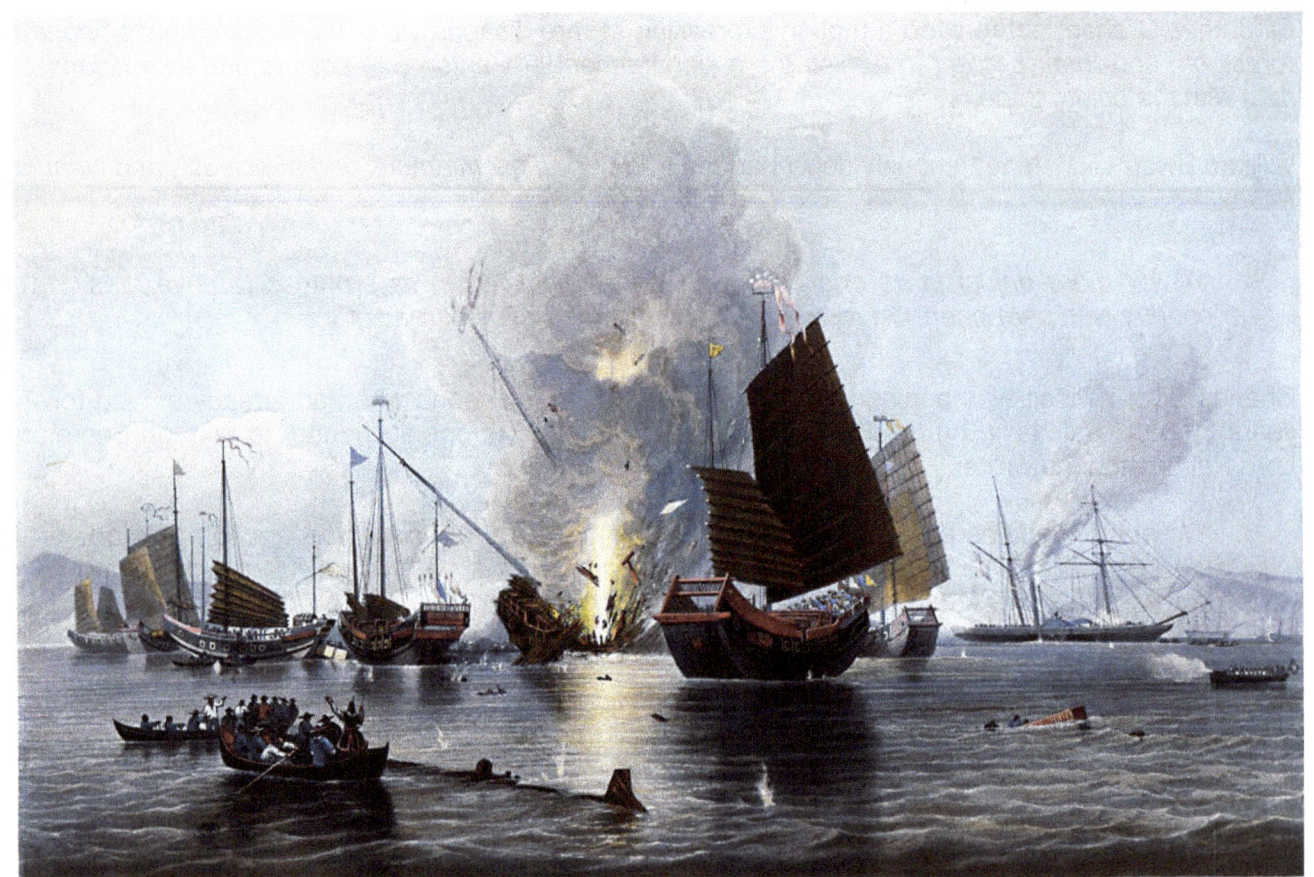

The East India Company iron steam ship *Nemesis*, by Edward Duncan, 1843

6.5 The Second Opium War

Tensions between the British and the Chinese escalated, and the British faced attacks from local Chinese. Their attempts to enter the city of Canton were frustrated, and it was felt that China had not honoured the terms of the treaty. The Qing government was preoccupied with dealing with the Taiping Rebellion (Tàipíng Tiānguó Yùndòng).

The Treaty of Wanghia (Wàngshà Tiáoyuē) had been signed with America, and the Treaty of Whampoa (Huángpǔ Tiáoyuē) had been signed with France. With the growth of Western Imperialism, other nations hoped to gain increased access to trade with China and expand their overseas markets.

In October 1856, the cargo ship *Arrow* was seized by Chinese marines in Canton on suspicion of piracy. It had previously been used by pirates but had since been captured and resold, and was registered as a British ship at Hong Kong.

Harry Parkes, the British consul in Canton contacted the Imperial Commissioner Ye Mingchen and demanded its release and an apology. Nine of the crew were released, but Ye refused to release the remaining three. They were finally released in December after the Battle of Canton (Guǎngzhōu Chéng Zhànyì).

The British response was delayed by a general election, and the Indian Mutiny. The United States and Russian rejected offers of alliance, but France joined the British on account of the execution of a French missionary in Guangxi (Guǎngxī). British and French forces captured Canton in late 1857. Russia sent an envoy to Hong Kong but did not send any military aid.

The United States joined the British and French later after a Chinese garrison shelled a United States Navy steamer, also aiding in the Battle of Taku Forts (Dì èr Cì Dàgūkǒu Zhī Zhàn).

The British House of Commons passed a resolution on the 3rd March 1857 stating:

> "That this House has heard with the concern of the conflicts which have occurred between the British and Chinese authorities on the Canton River; and, without expressing an opinion as to the extent to which the Government of China may have afforded this country cause of complaint respecting the non-fulfilment of the Treaty of 1842, this House considers that the papers which have been laid on the table fail to establish satisfactory grounds for the violent measures resorted to at Canton in the late affair of the Arrow, and that a Select Committee be appointed to inquire into the state of our commercial relations with China".

Those who had supported the resolution were criticised for lack of patriotism, and the debate that followed ended in the Parliament being dissolved. The handling of the Second Opium War had effectively brought down the British government. The resulting general election resulted in a larger majority for the Whig party, who were in favour of military action.

The Chinese went on to suffer a decisive defeat, and the resulting Treaty of Tientsin (Tiānjīn Tiáoyuē) ensured that Britain, France, Russia, and the United States had the right to establish embassies in Peking.

Additional ports were opened up for trade, incuding Niuzhuang (Yíngkǒu), Tamsui (Dànshuǐ), Hankou (Hànkǒu), and Nanking (Nánjīng).

All foreign vessels had the right to travel freely on the Yangtze River and travel in the internal regions of China, and China was to pay four million taels of silver to Britain, and two million to France.

The Treaty of Aigun (Àihún Tiáoyuē) gave Russia left bank of the Amur River (Hēilóng Jiāng), a territory of over 600,000 square kilometres (231,660 square miles), with all restrictions on trade across the border being lifted.

The Convention of Peking (Běijīng Tiáoyuē) gave Britain southern Kowloon (Jiǔlóng) and Stonecutters Island (Ángchuánzhōu). Britain would later gain the New Territories south of the Sham Chun River (Shēnzhèn Hé) on the 9th June 1898.

Russia gained the territory of Outer Manchuria around the Golden Horn Bay on the Sea of Japan where the city Vladivostok was founded.

The further opening of trade and lifting of restrictions effectively legalised the opium trade, and the treaties would later be referred to as 'the unequal treaties'.

Western Imperialism and its ideas about free trade and open markets, clashed with Qing China's sense of self-sufficiency and self-protection from the destabilising forces of the outside world, and the threat of rebellion from within.

China had been dragged into the modern world against its will. This was a devastating blow to China which became weakened and decentralised by conflicts, internal fragmentations, continued military defeats, and losses of territory and wealth, which ultimately brought about the collapse of the Qing and dynastic rule in China. This was the beginning of what would be called China's 'Century of humiliation'.

Life in the farms and villages of China remained hard, but the port cities were a world away. International trade increased, attracting a growing number of wealthy merchants and business people. Domestic opium production increased, and opium dens gradually appeared in cities like Shanghai to offer entertainment to sailors and wealthy merchants alike, from underground vice dens to the most high-class establishments in Asia.

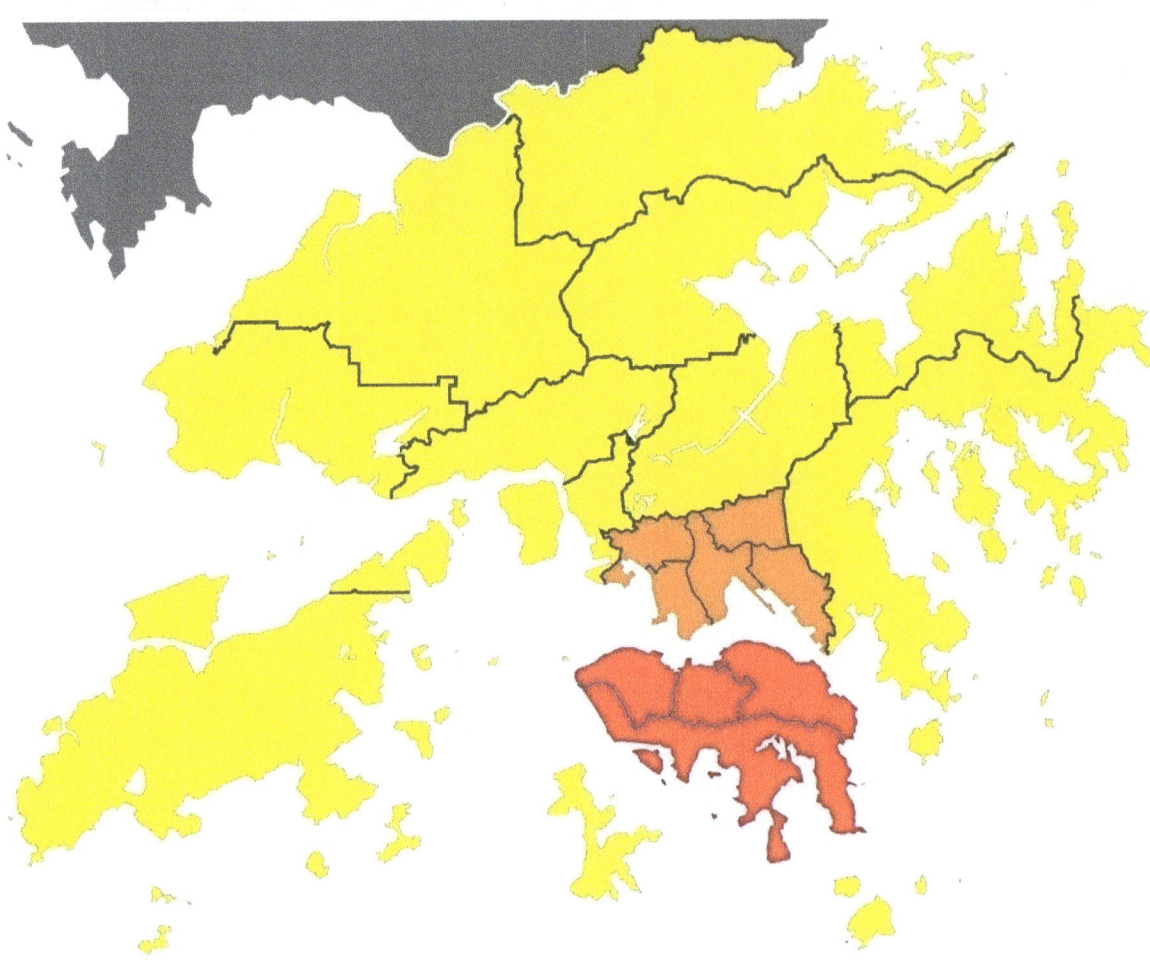

Hong Kong Island, Southern Kowloon, Stonecutter's Island, and the New Territories

MANCHURIA–U.S.S.R. BOUNDARY

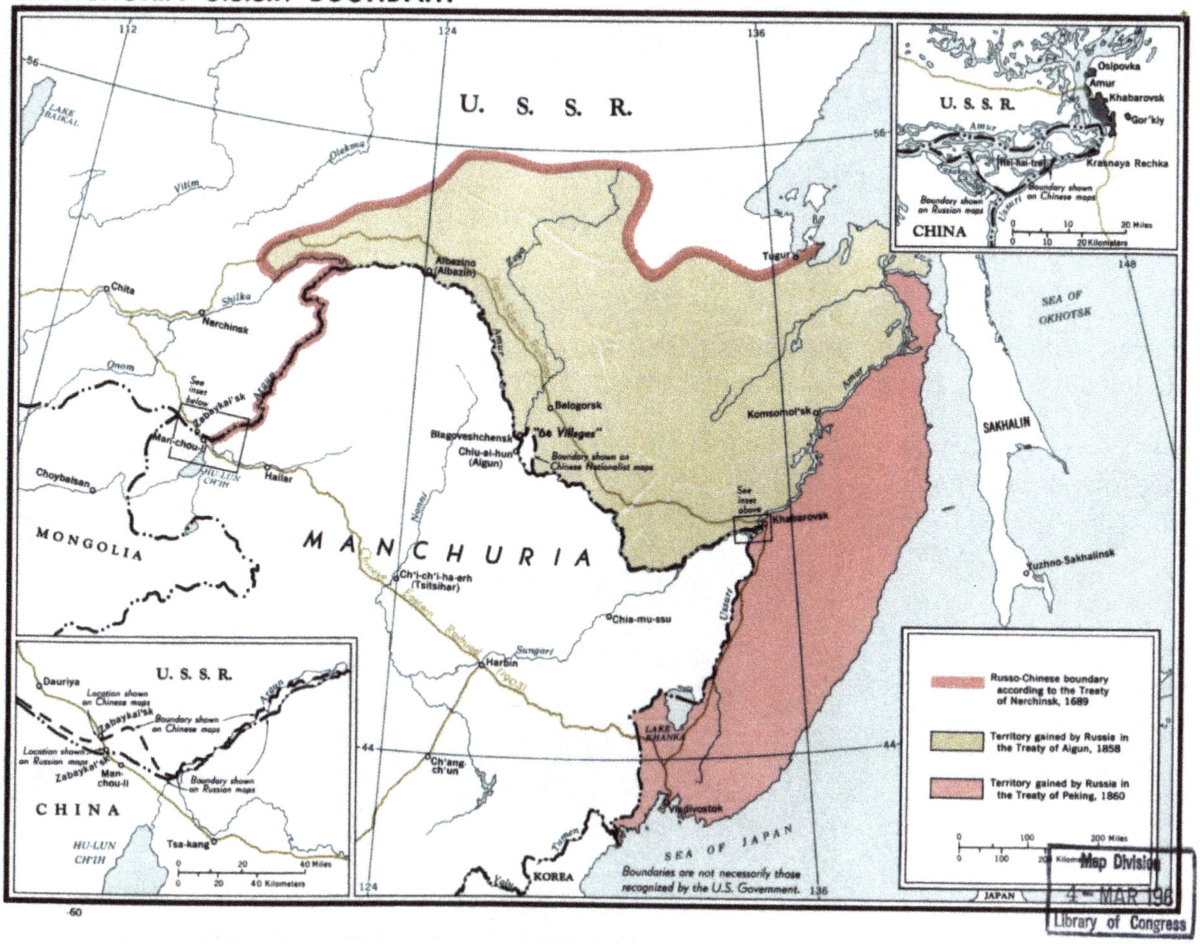

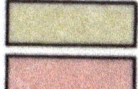

Russo-Chinese boundary according to the Treaty of Nerchinsk, 1689

Territory gained by Russia in the Treaty of Aigun, 1858

Territory gained by Russia in the Treaty of Peking, 1860

7. The 19th Century Part 2: *Danger, Addiction, and Vice (1850-1900)*

7.1 Science and 'God's Own Medicine'

Morphine was extensively used in the American Civil War (1861-1865) by medics who utilised its anaesthetic effects to perform increasingly prolonged surgical procedures, and it was also issued directly to soldiers as pain medication.

The Union Army alone used approximately 80 tons of opium tincture and powder and about 500,000 opium pills. During this time of the drug's popularity, users called opium 'God's own medicine'. Later it was found out that morphine was more addictive than either alcohol or opium.

The estimated number of soldiers in the American Civil War who were affected by the 'soldier's disease' of morphine addiction vary from 50,000 to 400,000. The use of opiates for general anesthesia began to be replaced by diethyl ether and chloroform, which was relatively safe compared to opiates.

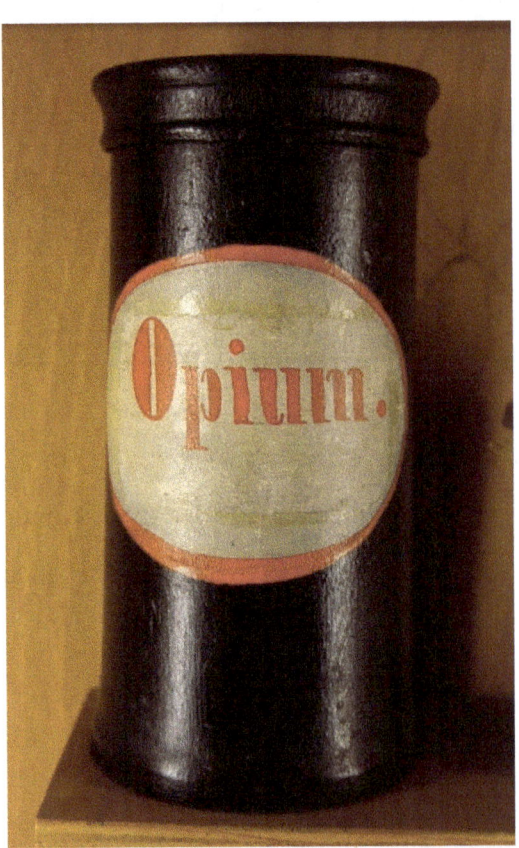

A vessel for the storage of pharmaceutical opium, c1800s

Alexander Wood (1817-1884) was a Scottish physician. He invented the first true hypodermic syringe in 1853. He referred to it as 'subcutaneous', and the term 'hypodermic' was invented by the English doctor Charles Hunter, who developed Wood's invention as a method of administering pain relief.

Charles R A Wright (1844-1894) was an English lecturer in chemistry and physics. He sought to find a non-addictive alternative to morphine. In 1874 he boiled morphine over a stove for several hours and produced a more potent form of morphine called either *'diacetylmorphine'*, *'morphine diacetate'*, or *'diamorphine'*.

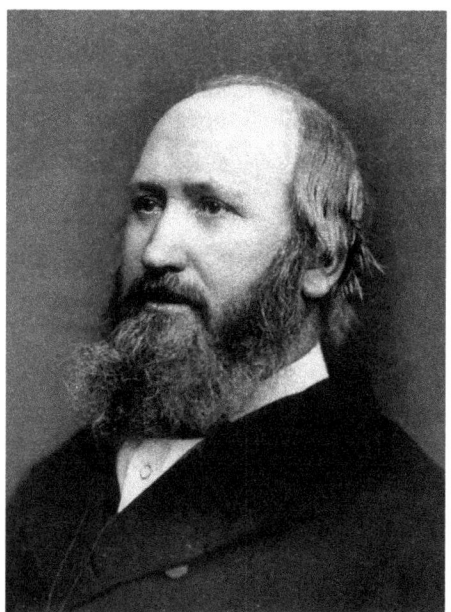
Alexander Wood, c1873

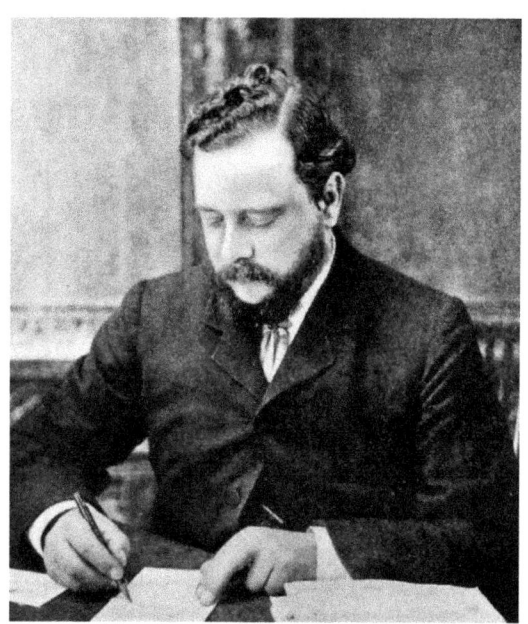
Charles R A Wright, c1876

Felix Hoffman (1868-1946) was a German chemist who worked at Bayer pharmaceutical company in Elberfeld, Germany. In the summer of 1897 he was instructed by his supervisor Heinrich Dreser to see if it was possible to synthesize codeine from morphine. Instead the experiment produced diamorphine which was about twice the strength of morphine. The head of Bayer's research department is said to have named the new drug '*heroin*' based on the German '*heroisch*' (heroic, strong, from the ancient Greek word '*heros*', '*ἥρως*').

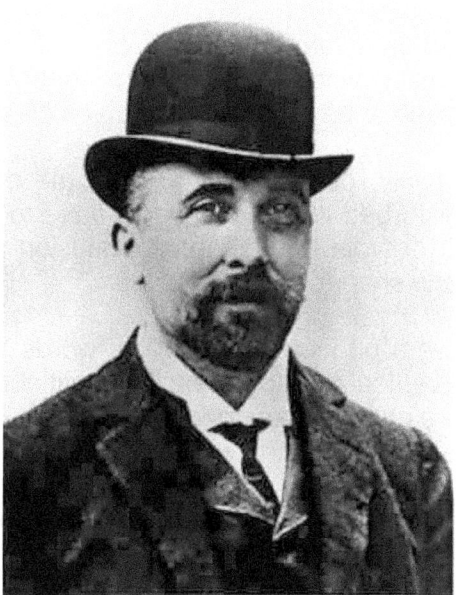
Felix Hoffman, date unknown

While not the first to make heroin, Bayer discovered ways in which to make it commercially, and in 1898 it was being marketed as an over-the-counter drug to treat coughs without the side-effects of morphine. Despite Bayer's advertising, heroin would soon have one of the highest addiction rates among users.

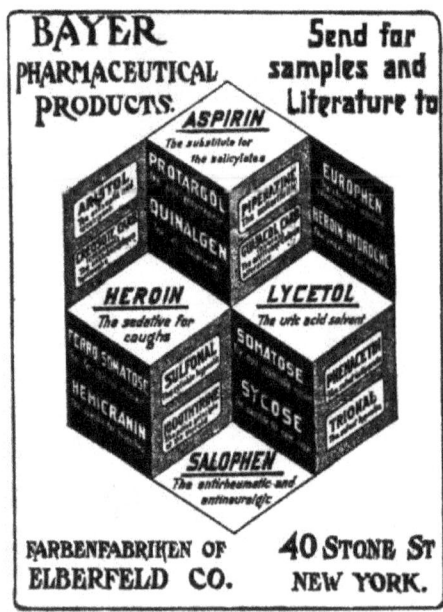

An advertisement for Bayer Pharmaceuticals, before 1904

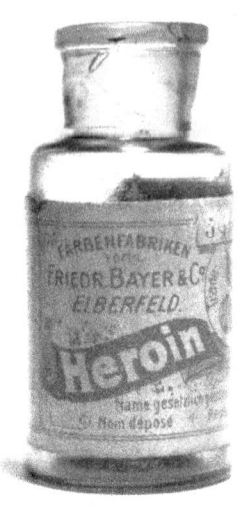

A Bayer heroin bottle

Another opiate available over-the-counter was called Paregoric, which appeared in the London Pharmacopoeia of 1721 under the name '*Elixir Asthmaticum*', and later in 'The Medical Companion, Or Family Physician' of 1827 as '*Paregoric Elixir*'.

It was originally developed by Jakob Le Mort (1650-1718) at Leiden University in the Netherlands. The word 'paregoric' comes from the Greek word '*parēgorikós*', meaning soothing, to console or comfort.

Similarly to laudanum, it was based on opium dissolved in alcohol, and it also contained benzoic acid, aniseed, honey, and camphor gum. It was widely used to control diarrhoea, as an expectant and cough medicine, to calm children, and to be rubbed on the gums of teething babies to soothe pain.

In an age without domestic electricity, people waking up in the middle of the night with ailments, complaints, and symptoms that disturbed their sleep would have to search their medicine cabinet by candlelight. For this reason, and to avoid any potential confusion and accidental poisoning, bottles were made in distinctive colours and shapes.

Cobalt blue and emerald green were popular choices. The words 'poison' or 'not to be taken' were also embossed on one side with vertical ribs to be easily identifiable to the touch. One chemist who used this design in the manufacture of their '*Paregoric Elixir*' was E. E. Hall & Co. of Wolverhampton in the West Midlands of England.

Despite the intention of such distinctive bottles giving a kind of visual warning, it was found that the distinctive colours and shapes of these bottles attracted curiosity in children.

There were also cases appearing in the news of people being deliberately poisoned by opiates and other dangerous substances readily available in any chemist, and it caused doctors and manufacturers to think again. In the beginning of the 20th century, regulation increased, and there were more and more restrictions about what could be sold and how it should be packaged, and these bottles were phased out.

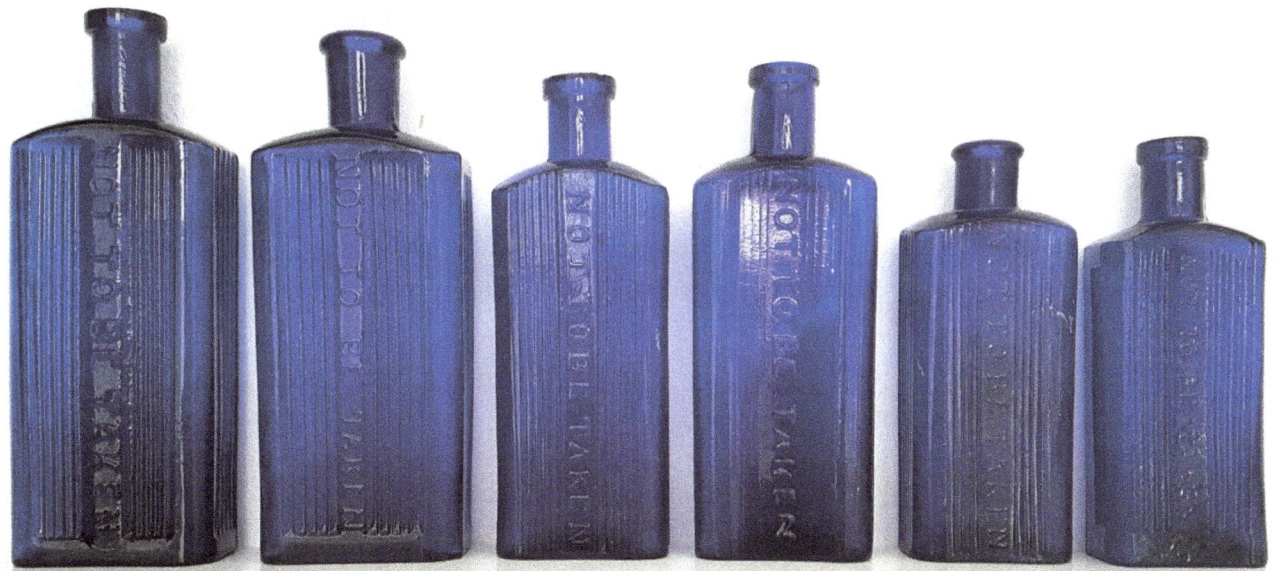
Vintage cobalt blue opiate bottles c1890-1910, 8oz, 6oz, and 3oz, author's collection

7.2 From East to West: The Spread of Opium Culture

Due to famine, political upheaval, and the rumours of a better life to be had outside of East and Southeast Asia, Chinese emigrants began to seek a better life in the West. The enclaves where the Chinese immigrant communities settled were nicknamed 'Chinatowns'. In the United States, San Francisco was the first point of entry for Chinese immigrants, some of whom hoped to participate in the California Gold Rush of 1848-1855, or to find work on the first Transcontinental Railroad.

The rituals and traditions of smoking opium that were widespread in their homeland were brought with them, including the establishments where opium was sold and smoked, the 'opium den'. Opium dens appeared in the Chinatowns of San Francisco and New York, and in Victoria and Vancouver in British Columbia, Canada. The Chinese people who ran the opium dens would have had access to a network of contacts to be able to procure the supply of all the required paraphernalia including pipes, lamps, tools, and opium, which would have been prepared by staff for first-timers and non-Chinese visitors.

Customers would recline on a purpose built bed and hold the prepared pipe over the opium lamp inhaling the vapours. People from all levels of society in China would visit opium dens. They varied in style from the most luxurious and opulent to the simplest spaces with sparse furnishings, reflecting the financial means of their customers.

In 1874 in San Francisco, smoking opium in the city limits was banned, and confined to neighbouring Chinatowns and their opium dens. Anti-Chinese sentiment grew with the perception that non-Chinese people were now frequenting the opium dens, and in 1875, the San Francisco Opium Den Ordinance banned them as follows:

> "No person shall maintain or visit, or shall in any way contribute to the support of any place, house, or room where opium is smoked".

The 47th Congress even went so far as to sign the Chinese Exclusion Act in 1882, banning Chinese immigration into the United States. This resulted in the so called 'driving out' period which led to large scale violence including The Rock Springs Chinese Massacre of 1885 and the Hells Canyon Massacre of 1887. The United States economy suffered a great loss as a result. Opium continued to be imported and was increasingly taxed from US$6 to US$300 per pound of opium, until the Opium Exclusion Act of 1909 banned it altogether.

The idea of opium dens being widespread in Victorian London are largely fictionalised, and invented by authors and journalists to satisfy a public demand for sensational stories of intrigue, danger, criminal underworlds, and a sense of the unknown lying around the corner. This included works such as Thomas Burke's '*Limehouse Nights*', Sax Rohmer's '*The Mystery of Dr. Fu-Manchu*', Charles Dickens's '*The Mystery of Edwin Drood*', and Sir Arthur Conan Doyle's Sherlock Holmes story '*The Man with the Twisted Lip*'.

By 1830 the demand for opium for medicinal and recreational uses in Britain had reached such heights that the small amount that could be produced in Britain was not enough, and so 9.8 tons of opium was imported in 157 chests from Turkey and India.

Benjamin Broomhall (1829-1911) was a British advocate of foreign missions. He became an active opponent of the opium trade and wrote two books to advocating for the banning of opium called 'Truth about Opium Smoking' and 'The Chinese Opium Smoker'. He lobbied the British Parliament continually, and in his last days he heard the news from his son Marshall read to him from The Times newspaper that an agreement had been signed ensuring the end of the opium trade in two years.

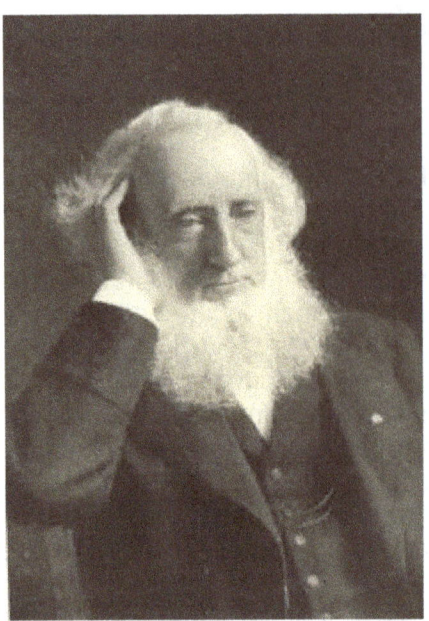

Benjamin Broomhall, date unknown

Another avenue for the arrival of opium dens in the West was in France. French expatriates returning home from colonies in French Indochina brought the practice back with them, and a large number of opium dens appeared in Marseille, Toulon, and Hyères. The New York Times of 27th April 1913 contained an article via special cable titled 'Opium Degrading the French Navy', that began as follows:

> *"PARIS, April 26--- A great outcry has arisen throughout the country over the serious revelations made by the well-known writer and duellist, Rouzier Dorcieres, concerning the hold that opium smoking has obtained on the French Navy in Southern seaports".*

From 1897 to 1902, Paul Doumer was Governor-General of French Indochina. The colonies were losing money, so the decision was made to tax various products, including opium. The Vietnamese, Cambodians and Laotians who couldn't or wouldn't pay the taxes lost their houses and land, forcing them to look for work as day labourers. This meant that France now had a financial interest in the continuation of the opium trade in Indochina.

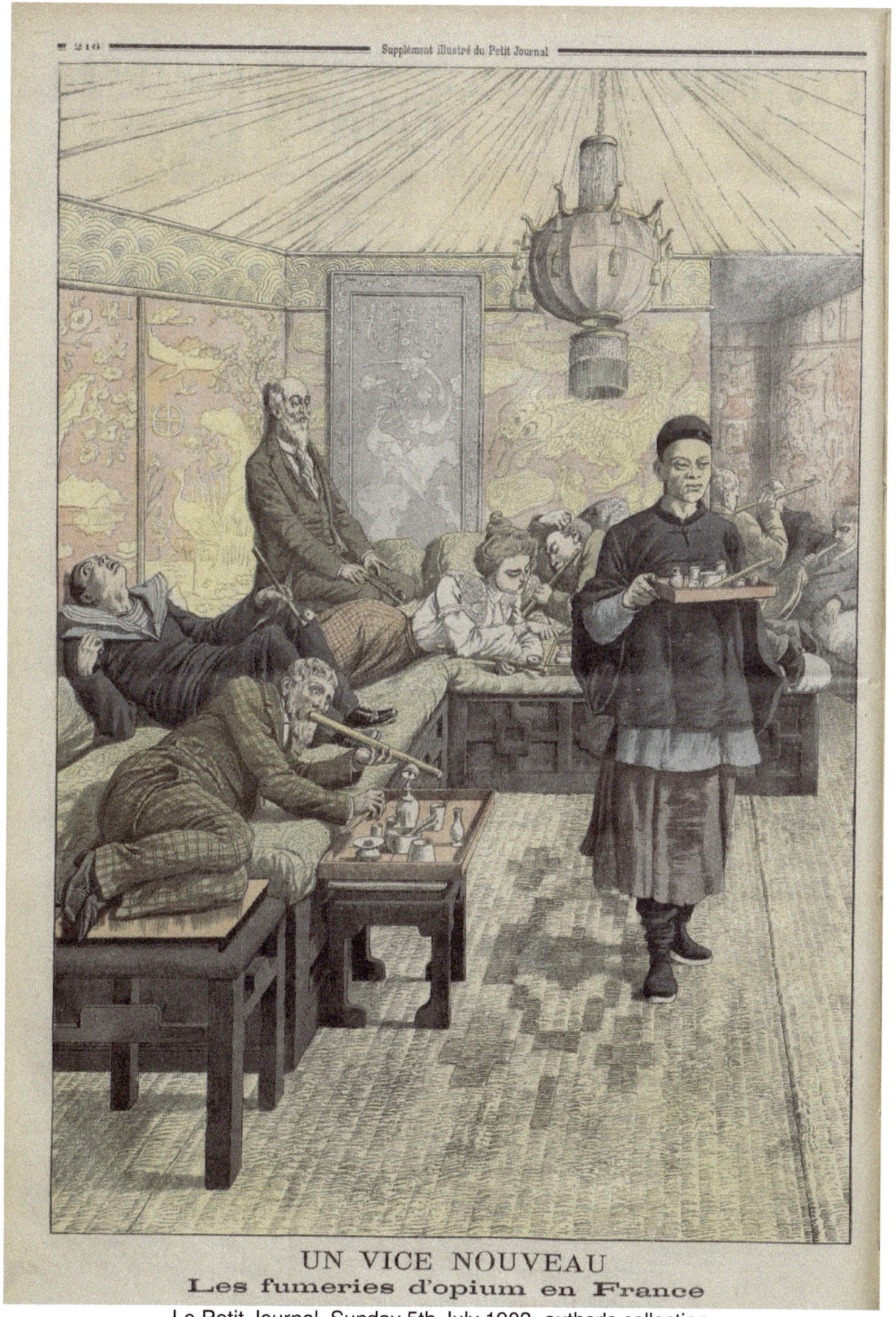

Le Petit Journal, Sunday 5th July 1903, author's collection

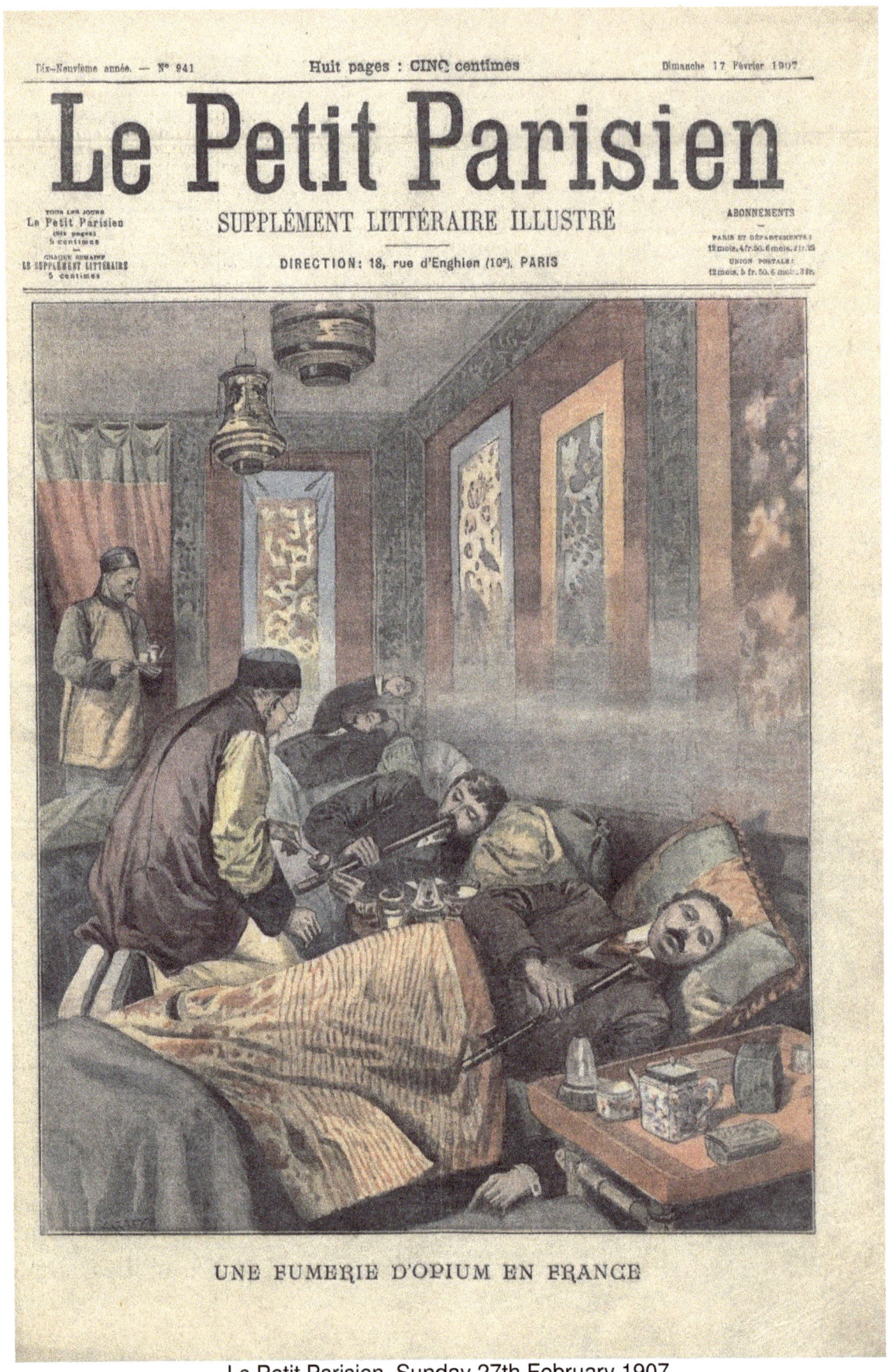

Le Petit Parisien, Sunday 27th February 1907
Gallica, digital library of the Bibliothèque nationale de France, public domain

7.3 Opium and Romanticism, Part 3

Charles Baudelaire (1821-1867) was a French poet. His collections of poetry: 'Les Fleurs du Mal' (The Flowers of Evil, 1857), 'Les Paradis Artificiels' (Artificial Paradises, 1860), and 'Les Spleen de Paris' (Paris Spleen, 1869), were groundbreaking and influential.

The tone of his work argued away from the earlier Romantics and their belief in the supremacy of nature, and instead focused on individual moral complexity, decadence, vice, and melancholy.

His health was plagued by illnesses, and by his smoking of opium and use of laudanum. The latter is referred to in his prose poem The Double Room, published in his collection 'Le Spleen de Paris' in 1869.

> *"In this narrow world, narrow but so full of disgust, a single object smiles at me: the phial of laudanum; an old and terrible friend; like all friends, alas! full of caresses and of treachery".*

His work was considered controversial, scandalous, and deliberately provocative in its time, but it was then later described as ahead of its time.

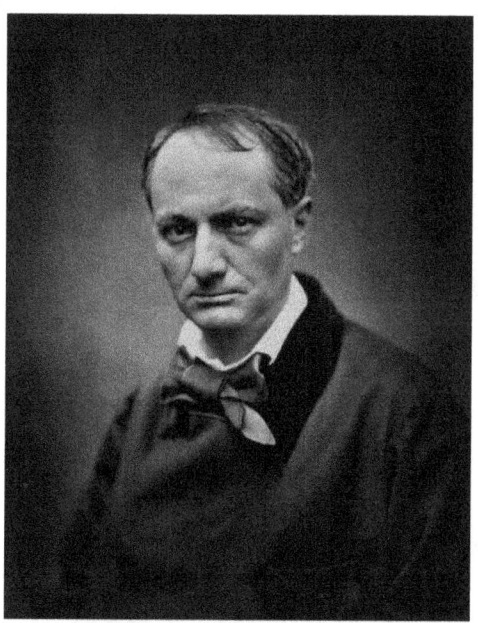
Charles Baudelaire, c1862

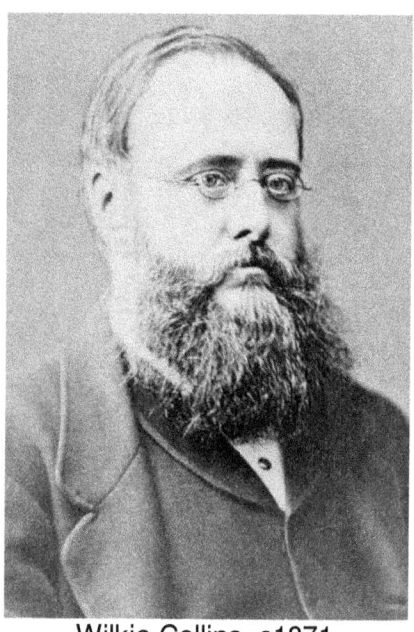
Wilkie Collins, c1871

Wilkie Collins (1824-1889) was an English novelist and playwright. In the 1860s he began to suffer from gout and became addicted to the opium he took for the pain. His experiences with the drug informed his treatment of them in his works, including a laudanum-addicted character in his novel Armadale of 1866, and also in 'The Moonstone' in 1868.

He created characters that were complex and believable, inviting the reader look past such obvious moral judgements that society made looking down at addicts, to explore the motivations and complex make-up of such characters, who are still capable of proving their morality despite substance dependence.

8. Modern Times: *Drugs, War, and Politics (1900-Present)*

8.1 Medicine and Addiction

At the beginning of the 20th century patent medicines containing opiates were still widely available over the counter for the treatment of bronchitis, diarrhoea, insomnia, nervous conditions, hysteria, and menstrual cramps. While they appeared to relieve the symptoms of many complaints, they cured very little. Debate grew within the medical community about how much heroin did actually treat ailments, or just mask the symptoms. For example respiratory ailments were being masked rather than treated because heroin depressed the respiratory system, reducing the impulse to cough.

The medical marketplace had not yet been regulated, and doctors and patients were tempted to overprescribe or overuse opiates. Medical journals published more and more warnings about the dangers to be avoided of opiate addiction, but due to a shortage of alternative options for treatment, the problem continued, creating more and more addicts.

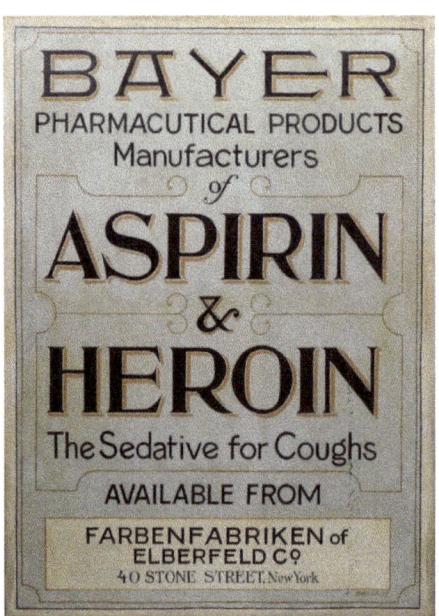

A replica of an advertising sign from Bayer for use in US drug stores before 1924

Heroin was still seen as a safer and non-addictive alternative to morphine, and it was even thought that it could be used to treat morphine addicts and help them to give up their habit. The Saint James Society in the US offered to supply morphine addicts with heroin through the post to help them give up their habit.

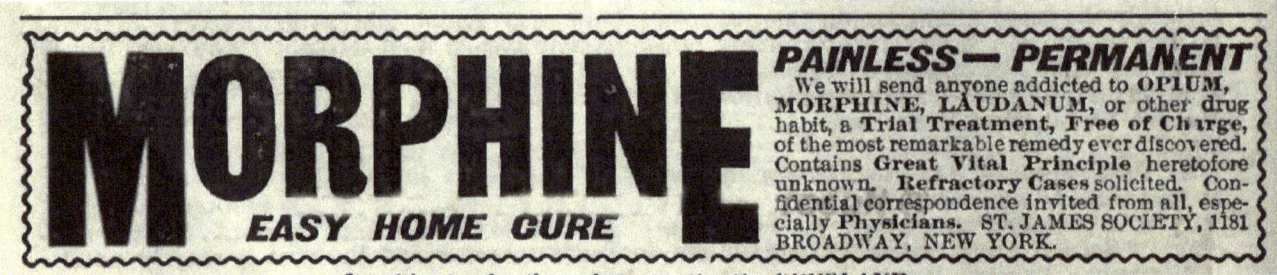

A newspaper advert offering a cure for Morphine by the Saint James Society, c1900

Advances in medicine resulted in a shift away from the use of opiates for general anaesthesia, and a greater knowledge and understanding of germs and diseases brought about improvements in public health, which resulted in fewer cases of dysentery or other gastrointestinal diseases, and fewer patients resorting to opiates to relieve their symptoms.

Soldiers in World War I turned to drugs in several ways, stimulants were used to combat fatigue, and opiates were used to treat pain and injuries, often being self-prescribed. The accepted recommended dose was 16 milligrams, but in the confusion and chaos, patients were sometimes given more than one dose, and those in severe pain were given larger amounts.

Some soldiers would often self-prescribe a dose before help could arrive, and morphine would be administered for weeks on end during the subsequent treatment and recovery of patients, and many developed addictions. It was even possible for the soldiers' loved ones to buy and send gift packs labelled as 'useful presents for our friends on the front' containing heroin and cocaine.

8.2   Regulation and Prohibition in the United States

Public criticism of the opium trade, the rise in drug abuse, and its affect on society brought about a growing anti-opium movement, particularly from religious groups. While politicians sought to crack down on the trade in opium, morphine, and heroin, the demand continued, forcing existing addicts to buy from illegal street dealers. The trade was forced underground, and a black market opened up.

In the United States, the Pure Food and Drink Act of 1906 required that any products containing addictive substances such as opium, morphine, or heroin must be labelled.

The Opium Exclusion Act of 1909 banned the importation of opium for smoking. Smugglers were arrested, contraband was confiscated, and raids were carried out on dealers and dens. This was designed to target opium smoking practised by Chinese immigrants, rather than the widely available over-the-counter opiate medicines.

Anti-Chinese sentiment continued to grow in the United States and Canada, and other places in the west where enclaves of Chinese immigrants had established Chinatowns, driven by the fear that an increasing number of non-Chinese citizens were frequenting opium dens.

Hamilton Wright (1867-1917) was an American physician and pathologist who was appointed as United States Opium Commissioner by US President Theodore Roosevelt and attended the International Opium Commission on the 26th February 1909 in Shanghai. This was one of the first steps towards international drug prohibition.

Wright was quoted in the New York Times in an article titled "Uncle Sam is the Worst Drug Fiend in the World" published on the 12th March 1911:

> "Of all the nations of the world, the United States consumes most habit-forming drugs per capita. Opium, the most pernicious drug known to humanity, is surrounded, in this country, with far fewer safeguards than any other nation in Europe fences it with".

The International Opium Convention signed at The Hague on the 23rd January 1912 was the first international treaty on drug control. It became effective on the 11th Feb 1915, and was incorporated into the Treaty of Versailles on the 28th June 1919.

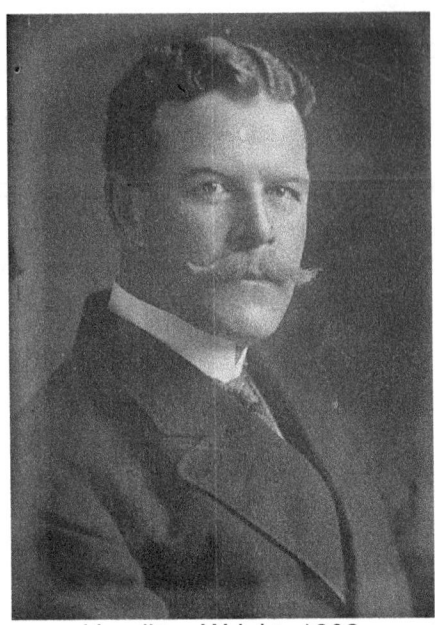
Hamilton Wright, 1909

In the United States, the Harrison Narcotics Tax Act of 1914 regulated and taxed the production, importation, and distribution of opiates for medicinal use, restricted the amount of opiates that could be used in medicines, and required a doctor's prescription for the use of such drugs.

On the 17th January 1920 in the United States, the Volstead Act came into effect with a federal ban on the production, importation, transportation, and sale of alcoholic beverages. Organised crime which had previously focused on gambling and prostitution saw the potential of profiting from the black market in alcohol, and the practice of 'bootlegging' (smuggling over land) and 'rum-running' (smuggling by sea) became organised and managed by criminal gangs, who frequently fought each other in violent clashes over territory.

On 26th May 1922 congress passed the Narcotic Drugs Import and Export Act to enforce the Harrison Act and to tightly oversee the import and export of opiates, to ban all recreational use, and to control the quality of what was being used for medical purposes. As the profitability of the black market increased and operations expanded, more and more police officers and politicians were bribed to offer political protection, and more men were recruited and armed to protect the transportation and storage of alcohol, not only from federal agents, but rival gangs.

The US Federal Burea of Narcotics (FBN) was formed in 1930 to enforce the Harrison Narcotics Act of 1914, the Narcotic Drugs Import and Export Act of 1922, and to combat opium and heroin smuggling. Offices were opened up in France, Italy, Turkey, Beirut, and Thailand. Federal agents cooperated with local drug enforcement authorities gathering intelligence on smugglers and made undercover busts locally.

On the 20th February 1933 the Blaine Act was used to repeal the Volstead Act, returning the control of alcohol to state and local level. With the black market for alcohol drying up, organised crime groups shifted their focus towards other practices, such as the opium trade.

8.3 Regulation and Prohibition in Britain

The British government passed the Poisons and Pharmacy Act of 1908, and introduced further regulations under the Defence of the Realm Act 1914 (abbreviated to DORA). Regulation 40B made illegal the sale of opium-based products and cocaine to military personnel without prescription, except for medical practitioners.

In February 1916, pharmacies in London were fined for failing to observe the restrictions of the Pharmacy Act of 1908 when selling morphine to military men. The Army Council issued an order banning any unauthorised sale or supply of opium, morphine, and heroin to any member of the armed forces, except for medical reasons and only by prescription.

The Dangerous Drugs Act of 1920 kept much of the detail of DORA regulation 40B, taking regulation away from pharmacists, and away from a wartime emergency measure to a permanent peacetime law applying to all citizens. There was some disagreement about whether the Ministry of Health or the Home Office should be given overall control. The Home Office was favoured, which was seen by some as symbolising the priority of punishment over a medical approach to the drug problem.

8.4 Regulation and Prohibition in China

By 1905 an estimated 25% of the male population of China were regular consumers of opium. In 1906 Chinese resistance to opium was stepped up with a new initiative aiming to eliminate the drug problem within 10 years. In 1908 Britain agreed to reduce opium imports into China by 10% per year in return for China also reducing its domestic production.

In China there were mass meetings where opium paraphernalia was publicly burned, and public opinion was turned against opium and its users. This effort was short-lived however and after the death of Yuan Shikai in 1916, the Chinese political system fragmented into what would be called the 'Warlord Era' (Jūnfá shídài). The warlords used opium as a revenue source, selling the rights to grow and sell opium within their provinces. The most infamous of whom was Zhang Zongchang, who the former Puyi Emperor described as "

> "a universally detested monster"... "tinged with the livid hue induced by heavy opium smoking".

8.5 Organised Crime in the United States: The Commission

The Five Families of New York   The Chicago Outfit   The Buffalo Family

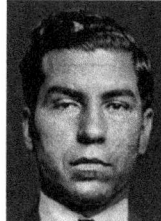
Charlie 'Lucky' Luciano

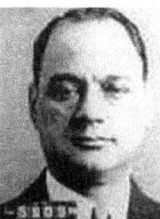
Vincent Mangano

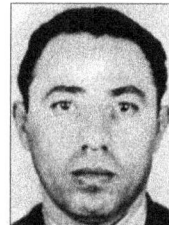
Tommy Gagliano

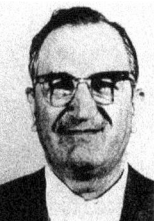
Joseph Bonnano

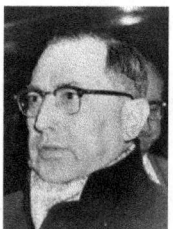
Joe Profaci

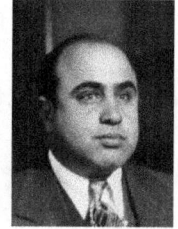
Al Capone

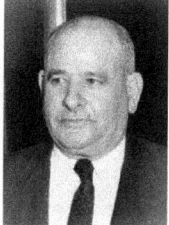
Stefano Magaddino

The entrepreneurial criminal minds who seized the opportunity to profit from the Prohibition Era transformed the criminal underworld from one of loose gangs of thugs into one of big business, managed like a joint association, based on capitalist principles, supplying a demand that was profitable though illegal. They were mainly made up of people from the Italian-American Mafia, the Jewish Mob, and to a lesser degree, members of the Irish Mob, and African-American organised crime groups. They put aside traditional reservations about which criminal community their associates were from, so long as there was money to be made. After the Castellammarese War, Charlie 'Lucky' Luciano called a meeting in Chicago to resolve the situation, and a governing body called 'The Commission' was formed to coordinate criminal activity across the United States.

Instead of acting under the title of '*capo di tutti capi*' (boss of all bosses) he instead chose to maintain a quiet power over all of the families. He acted as chairman over a 'board of directors' who would meet every five years, or when needed, to mediate conflicts between them to prevent any further gang wars, as they were costly and bad for business. This level of organisation led to an increase in the supply and demand for morphine and heroin.

The United States government struck a deal with Lucky Luciano and the Commission of organised crime families to assist the US Navy with its intelligence gathering. They were also tasked with preventing any strikes or sabotage, protecting against black market theft of vital war supplies and equipment, and reporting any attempts by German or Italian agents to enter the waterfront.

Luciano was also able to strike a deal with the US Government to provide intelligence, contacts, and local assistance to help pave the way for the Allied invasion of Sicily in 1943. Luciano's mafia connections were happy to see Benito Mussolini toppled since he had cracked down hard on the mafia and its activities.

During World War II the opium trade had ground to a halt. Distribution routes were blocked, the flow of opium was cut off, and the number of addicts in the United States fell to a record low of 20,000.

8.6 Organised Crime in Europe: The Corsican Mafia

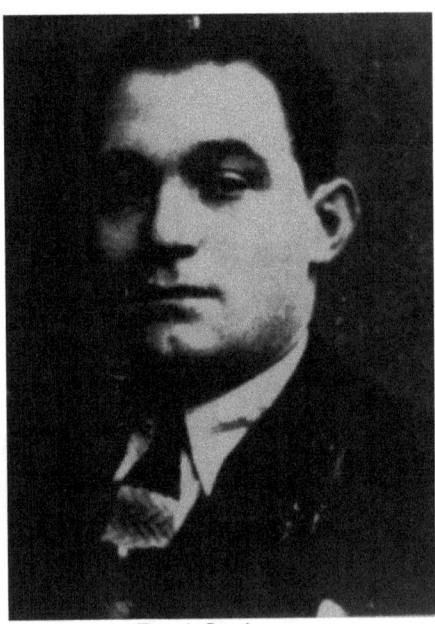
Paul Carbone

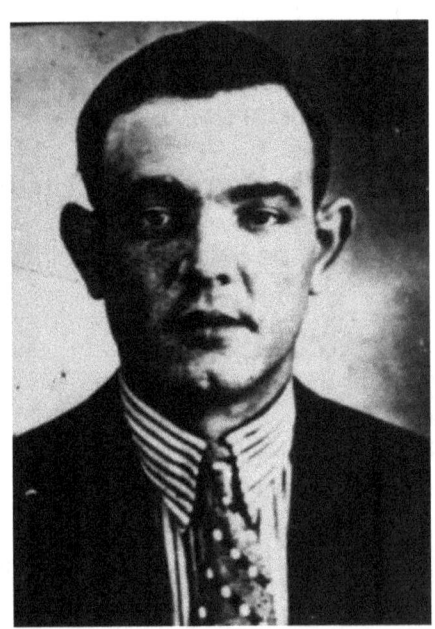
François Spirito

The heroin laboratories owned and operated by the Corsican mafia were discovered near Marseille in 1937. Marseille was one of the busiest ports in the Mediterranean, and with so many ships passing through every day, shipments of heroin were difficult to detect.

After World War II, the United States CIA (Central Intelligence Agency) and the French *Service de Documentation Extérieure et de Contre-Espionnage* (External Documentation and Counter-Espionage Service) commonly referred to as the SDECE, protected the Corsican mafia in return for their protection and control of the Old Port of Marseille to prevent French communists taking over. In the few years that followed, members of the Corsican mafia found their way into elected political office, some served in the Gendarmarie (Military Police), and some in the SDECE itself.

France was keen to keep hold of its colonies in Indochina after World War II, and to maintain their profitability. The Hmong people in North Vietnam and Laos had been encouraged to increase their opium production. The SDECE were able to use proceeds from the opium trade to fund their operations in the Indochina War to resist communist insurgency.

In 1954, following a disastrous defeat in the battle of 'Dien Bien Phu', the French were forced to withdraw from Indochina. Vietnam was partitioned along the 17th parallel, with the Democratic Republic of Vietnam in the north, and the State of Vietnam in the south. The Corsican mafia flew drugs from Laos to South Vietnam by plane from then on, the operations were collectively known as 'Air Opium'.

8.7 Organised Crime in China: The Green Gang

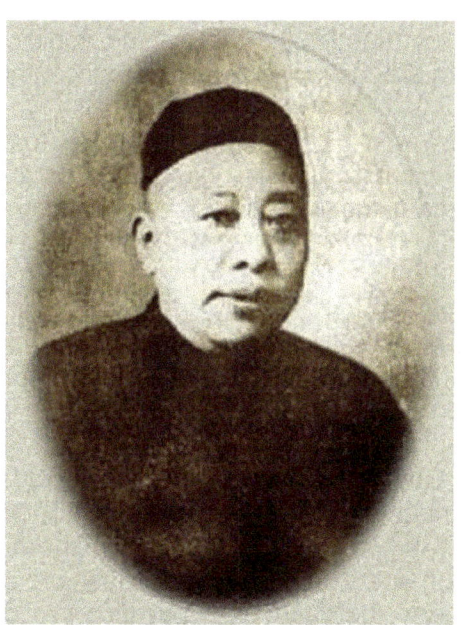
Huang Jinrong

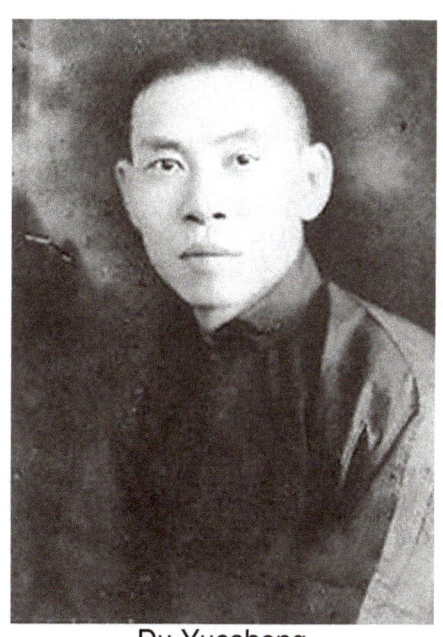
Du Yuesheng

In the 1920s and 1930s most of the heroin that was smuggled into the United States was produced in China and refined in Shanghai. Trade was managed by Huang Jinrong, Du Yuesheng, and other members of the Green Gang (*Qīng Bāng*). Because of the different jurisdictions and administrations in Shanghai, the legal process was complicated, and these complications served as obstacles to law enforcement and allowed organised crime to flourish.

The ruling nationalist Kuomintang of the Republic of China not only faced a growing insurgency by the Chinese Communist Party, but also invasion and occupation by the Empire of Japan, which became part of the wider theatre of the War in the Pacific during World War II. After the Japanese formally surrendered on the 2nd September 1945, the Chinese Civil War continued, concluding in 1949 with the victory of the Chinese Communist Party and the establishment of the People's Republic of China led by Chairman Mao Zedong.

The Mao Zeodong government eradicated opium production and consumption in China, with ten million addicts forced into compulsory treatment. Dealers were executed, and opium-producing regions were planted with new crops. Opium production shifted to Southeast Asia, and the defeated Chinese Nationalist Kuomintang (KMT) retreated to Taiwan and Burma.

8.8 Southeast Asia and the Golden Triangle

Southeast Asia lay between the major maritime routes from India to China, and became part of the expanding Asian opium trade as a significant secondary market for both Indian and Chinese opium production.

The profitability of opium became a major factor in Southeast Asia's modernisation. The business made up between 14% (Thailand) and 58% (British Malaya) of all tax revenues. Legal state-owned monopolies of over 6,000 licensed opium dens, saw over 250 tons of opium supplied to over half a million registered smokers.

By the end of World War II, Southeast Asia was still an insignificant producer of opium, harvesting around 15 tons a year. At this time the supply of opium from India was relatively cheap, and so increased domestic cultivation was not seen as necessary.

It was not until the 1950s that pressure to end the opium trade brought about the abolition of opium dens by Southeast Asian governments, after which opium production increased significantly.

The work of the US Federal Bureau of Narcotics (FBN) was often frustrated by US foreign policy, particularly in Southeast Asia, where small scale Vietnamese smugglers were targeted and linked to resistance movements in South Vietnam, while investigations involving large scale smugglers in Thailand, which was a US ally, were inconclusive.

Information on the size and complexity of the Southeast Asian drug trade had not yet been fully obtained even by the 1960s. In March 1965, the FBN compiled a list of 246 international drug traffickers, only two of which were listed as active in Southeast Asia, and these were members of the Corsican Mafia.

Fear of the 'Domino Effect' of communism expanding in Southeast Asia caused the United States and France to give their covert support to various warlords, tribes and militia in the Golden Triangle region, providing them and their armies with logistical support, ammunition, and arms in the fight against communist forces, and also air transport for the production and sale of their main cash crop of opium. The doctrine of 'indirect intervention' created local allies in the Cold War, but also brought about a series of consequences that it had not predicted.

8.9 The French Connection

Opium produced in the region went on to supply a major smuggling scheme that would become known as 'The French Connection'. Raw opium was transported from Southeast Asia, and also later Turkey, to laboratories operated by the Corsican mafia in Marseille, France, where it was refined into heroin and shipped to the American Continent.

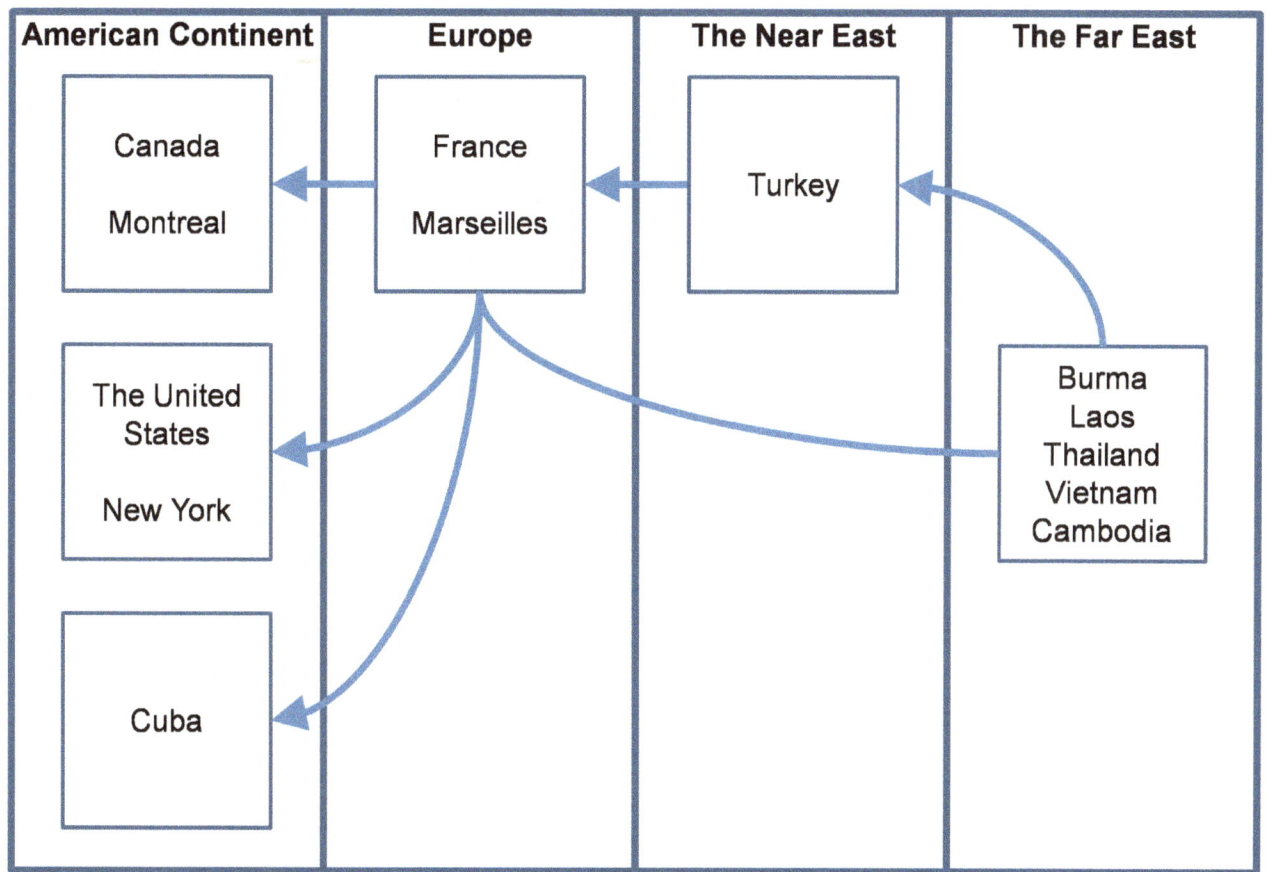

Burma had been a colony of the British Empire since 1824. It had first been ruled as a province of British India, and then in 1935 it was given the status of a separate colony in its own right. The Japanese occupation of Burma in World War II destabilised British rule in the area, leading to Burmese independence in 1948. Communist insurgencies began soon afterwards.

After the Chinese Communist Revolution of 1949, the forces of the Chinese Nationalist Kuomintang (KMT) in the south east were evacuated to Taiwan, and in the south west were driven out of the Yunnan province of China into the Shan states of northeast Burma. The KMT hoped to use the territory as a refuge to regroup, resupply, and retrain, and then as a base to mount further attacks to retake China.

The CIA backed the approximately 14,000 KMT soldiers as an allied anti-communist force, which from their location could gather intelligence and monitor for signs of a possible Chinese advance into Southeast Asia, and also open up a second front in the Korean War against North Korea and China.

With the approval of US President Harry Truman the CIA transported weapons to the KMT in Burma from the KMT stronghold in Taiwan, via Thailand with the approval of Thailand's Prime Minister Plaek Phibunsongkhram.

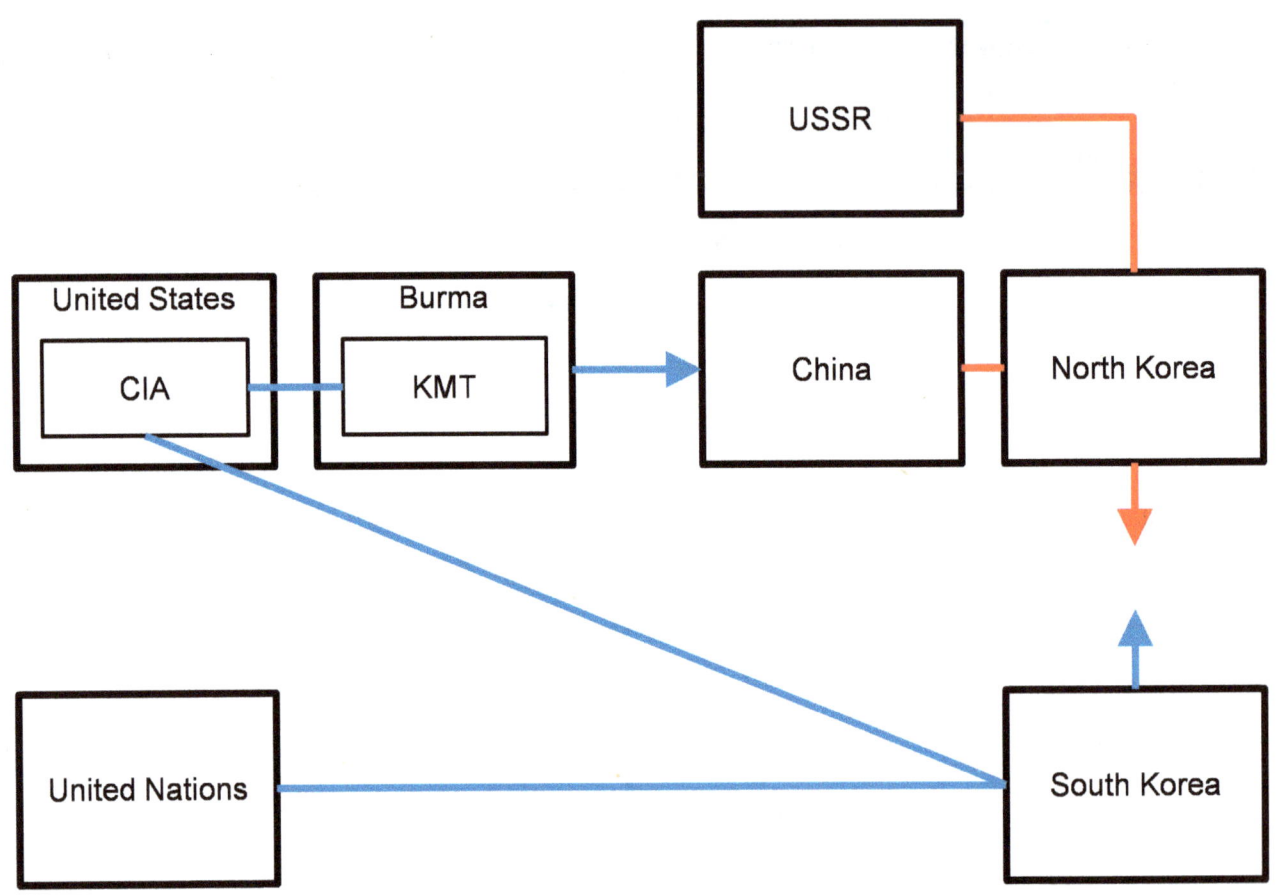

Three offensives followed, but they were ultimately defeated by the Chinese People's Liberation Army (PLA) and driven back with heavy losses each time. The KMT never invaded China again and instead chose to settle in the Shan states, a major opium-producing region.

The KMT dominated and controlled the opium-producing region and heavily taxed the production of opium, forcing local farmers to increase production to make ends meet. Annual production increased from 30 tons from 1948 to 600 tons by the mid 1950s. The KMT were eventually driven out of the Shan State of Burma in 1961, settling in northern Thailand.

An alliance with Thailand resulted in weapons and military supplies being exchanged for opium transported to Chiang Mai. From Chiang Mai the powerful police commander, and client of the CIA, General Phao Sriyanond shipped the opium south to Bangkok for local consumption and export. This paved the way for the subsequent private narcotic armies that emerged in the 'Golden Triangle' region.

One of the most powerful drug lords in the Shan state of Burma was Khun Sa. He had been given basic military training by the KMT in his youth, but gathered his own force of men and then became independent of the KMT.

He had been permitted by the Burmese government to use land to grow opium, in return for fighting against local rebels in the Shan state. The Burmese government hoped that the various drug lords would use proceeds from the opium trade to be self-supporting.

However, they used their profits to buy large supplies of military equipment from the black markets of Laos and Thailand, and were soon even better equipped than the Burmese army.

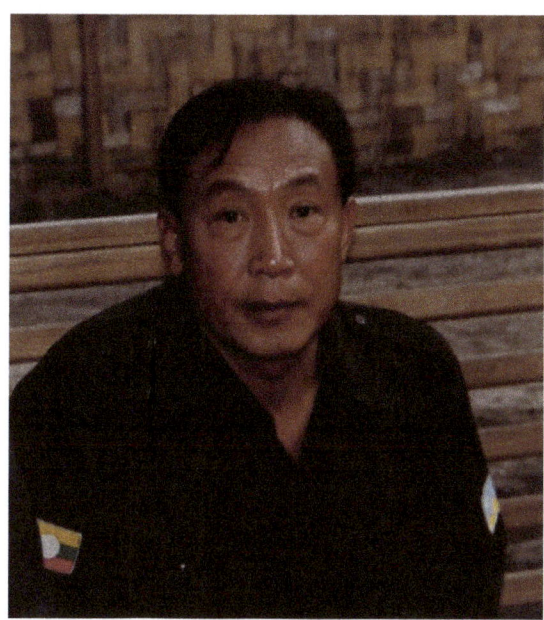

Khun Sa

The increase in profit and wealth from opium increased the rivalry between various warlords and armies to compete for dominance in the trade, which increased the need to protect cargo and personnel with more and more weaponry, making the region notoriously dangerous.

Laos had been a French colony since 1893, in which the Hmong people of the north had been encouraged to expand their opium production to increase the profitability of the colony. Opium had become their biggest and most important cash crop, which made up 15% of government revenues.

After the French withdrew from Indochina after defeat in the First Indochina War in 1954, the CIA moved in to support Laos against insurgency by communist forces, thereby inheriting the complex series of covert alliances and their indirect involvement in opium trading.

General Vang Pao was a native Hmong, and the only member of the Hmong community to rise to the rank of General in the Royal Lao Armed Forces. The United States government and intelligence community identified him as a potentially valuable ally and asset in the fight against communist insurgency.

Under French rule he had held command of the *Groupement de Commandos Mixtes Aéroportés* (Mixed Airborne Commando Group) commonly referred to as the GCMA. This was the 'Action Service' arm of the French *Service de Documentation Extérieure et de Contre-Espionnage* (External Documentation and Counter-Espionage Service) commonly referred to as the SDECE.

With CIA support, General Vang Pao maintained a private army of some 30,000 Hmong tribesmen in the north of Laos. The CIA provided assistance, military advisors, logistics, weapons, transportation, training in unconventional warfare, and later troops to fight against the communist Pathet Lao and the PAVN, with additional support from Thai and South Vietnamese forces. This private army was known as the 'Secret Army', and the Laotian Civil War would come to be known as the 'Secret War'.

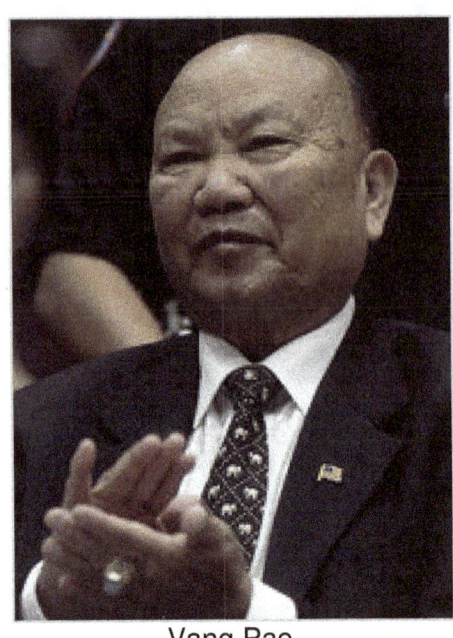

Vang Pao

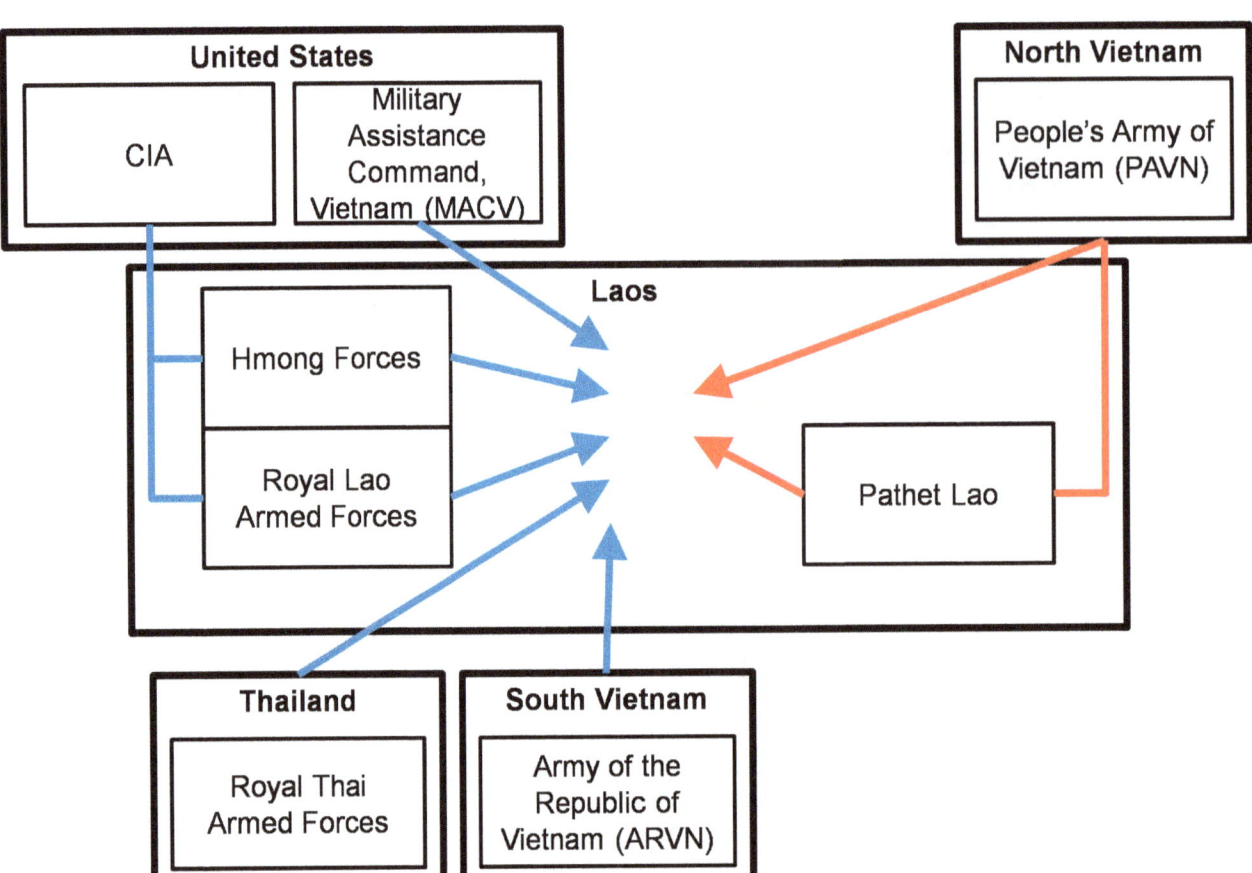

The so-called Opium War of 1967 occurred in Laos in July and August 1967 when the Burmese militia 'Shan United Revolutionary Army' (SURA) led by Khun Sa attempted to transport 16 tons of opium by mule to Royal Lao Army General Ouane Rattikone in Laos.

Because of earlier disagreements between the SURA and rival KMT regarding taxes for shipments of opium travelling through their neighbouring territory, as soon as the mule train crossed into Laos, it was attacked by KMT forces led by General Li Mi.

General Ouane Rattikone bombed both sides of the fighting, and then moved in troops to sweep the battlefield, and with both the SURA and the KMT defeated and expelled from Laos, he confiscated the opium for himself.

Following this conflict, the resulting bad publicity of the KMT brought about a Thai crackdown on all the KMT forces on their northern border, the KMTs revenue from the opium trade was diminished. Meanwhile in Burma, Khun Sa's attempt to gain a monopoly of the opium trade had failed. His army was defeated and humiliated and began to desert him, and his military strength declined.

Now that General Ouane Rattikone had obtained this supply of raw opium base, he had Chinese chemists flown in from Hong Kong to help improve his opium refineries. Rather than selling raw opium for refinement elsewhere into heroin, it could now be refined in-house and sold direct to the heroin market.

As well as being shipped worldwide, the heroin that had been produced in Laos was now being shipped to South Vietnam and sold to US forces in Vietnam who were their allies. In 1965 the Chinese Premier Zhou Enlai declared that the Chinese were encouraging opium consumption among troops in Vietnam in revenge for the Opium Wars.

8.10 CAT and Air America

Civil Air Transport (CAT) was set up by in 1946 by the American military aviator Claire Chennault and Whiting Willauer as a volunteer force known as the 'Flying Tigers' airlifting supplies and food into war-ravaged China using surplus World War II aircraft.

Under contract with the Chinese Nationalist KMT government, and later the CIA, efforts were soon diverted to assisting Chiang Kai-Shek and the KMT by flying supplies and ammunition to their forces on the Chinese mainland. With the defeat of the KMT in the Chinese Communist Revolution of 1949, CAT planes evacuated thousands of Chinese to Taiwan.

In August 1950, the CIA bought out Chennault and Willauer continuing to operate as CAT, eventually renaming the company 'Air America' in 1959. Air America inserted and extracted people including special forces, civilians, diplomats, spies, refugees, commandos, sabotage teams, doctors, war casualties, drug enforcement officers, and visiting VIPs such as Richard Nixon.

They flew photo reconnaissance missions which provided valuable intelligence on the activities of the Viet Cong, Pathet Lao, and the NVA. Their civilian marked aircraft were used under the control of the United States Air Force to launch search and rescue missions for downed pilots, and thousands of tons of food and livestock was flown in to support local tribes, including as live chickens, pigs, water buffalo, and cattle.

The Pathet Lao captured the Plain of Jars in 1964, which meant that the Royal Lao Air Force were unable to land their C-47 transport aircraft on the Plain of Jars. The Royal Laotian Air Force had almost no light planes that could land on the dirt runways near the mountaintop poppy fields. Having no way to transport their opium, the Hmong people were faced with economic ruin.

Vang Pao was given control over air drops of rice into the Hmong villages north and east of the Plain of Jars, and the air shipment of opium out of those Hmong villages to his headquarters in the so-called 'Secret City' of Long Tieng, also known as *Lima Site 98* (LS 98), or *Lima Site 20A* (LS 20A). With control of the two key commodities of rice and opium, Vang Pao became a powerful figure in Laos, and a hero of the Hmong people.

Allegations against Air America ranged from indirect complicity, tolerance, 'turning a blind eye', studied ignorance, profiting from, or actively participating in the opium trade. Responses to these allegations deny that any American owned airlines ever knowingly transported any opium, or that any American pilots every profited from any transporting of opium, and while only large items were checked, it may have been possible for some small amounts of opium to have found their way through unknown.

8.11 The War on Drugs

US involvement was Vietnam was blamed for the surge in illegal heroin being smuggled into the States, and an increase in the availability of heroin on the streets. On the 1st July 1973, President Richard Nixon created the Drug Enforcement Administration (DEA) to enforce federal drug laws and drug control activities.

In Turkey, there were opium farmers registered with the Turkish government to produce opium for medicinal purposes. Surplus opium was then sold on the black market, which found its way into the 'French Connection'.

The establishment of the DEA shifted the focus away from chasing drugs on the streets to attacking the source. Turkey was a poorer NATO ally under the shadow of the USSR at the height of the cold war, and in return for $35 million in aid, the poppy fields were eradicated. This looked like an early victory in the War on Drugs. However, Turkey was not the only source of raw opium. The shortfall in opium as a result of this action led to an increase in price, which increased incentives for production.

The next stage of the War on Drugs involved sending federal agents to Bangkok, Thailand. In cooperation with Thai police forces there were many seizures of heroin bound for the United States, which increased the risk of exporting to the United States to prohibitive levels. The market reacted by exporting instead to Europe, and Australia.

Mexican heroin appeared to fill the gap in the United States market left by the departure of Southeast Asian heroin. However, its supply was erratic, and its quality was inconsistent and nowhere near as well refined, which led to it being nicknamed 'Mexican Mud'.

The US and Mexican governments eliminated the source of 'Mexican Mud' by spraying poppy fields with Agent Orange. The amount detected in the US drug market declined, and so the operation was deemed successful.

8.12 The Golden Crescent

In response to the decrease in availability of 'Mexican Mud', another source of heroin was found in the 'Golden Crescent' area, including Iran, Afghanistan and Pakistan, creating an increase in the production and trade of illegal heroin.

Afghanistan and Pakistan had no opium production or consumption in the 1970s, but by 1981 Pakistan had become the world's largest producer of heroin, responsible for 60% of the supply to the United States. Pakistan had gone from having no heroin addicts to 5,000 by 1980, and over a million by 1985.

In 1978 the Soviet backed People's Democratic Party of Afghanistan (PDPA) took power in an event called the Saur Revolution. It began a series of modernisation and land reforms which were deeply unpopular with the traditional and rural population. Opposition was vigorously suppressed and thousands of political prisoners were executed. Anti-government armed groups emerged and large parts of the country were in open rebellion. The Soviet Union invaded Afghanistan in December 1979 to assist the PDPA in putting down the rebellion, beginning the Soviet-Afghan war.

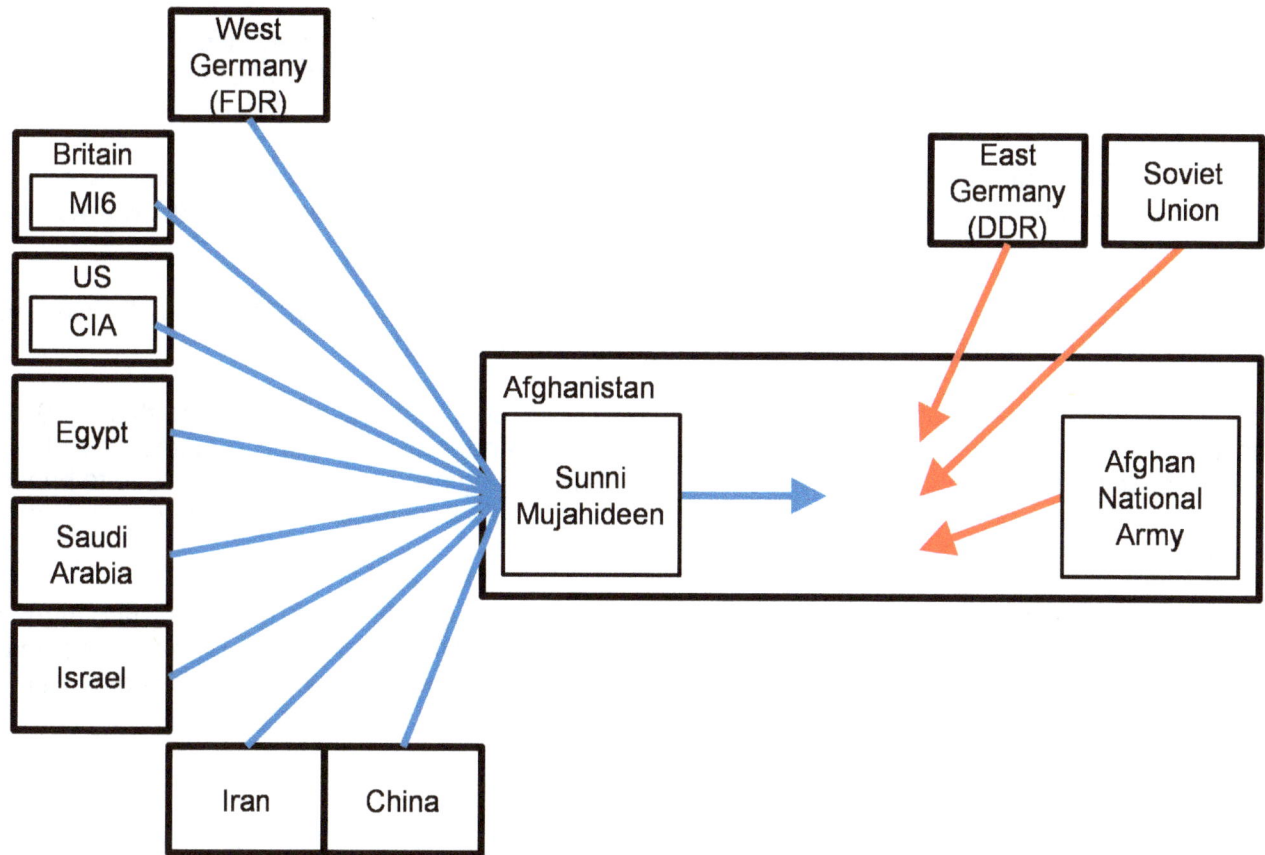

The CIA and MI6 covertly provided the Mujahideen with military advisors, training, supplies, and weapons. As they gradually liberated areas in Afghanistan, the Afghan guerrillas instructed their supporters to grow opium to fund the resistance, paying a portion of their crop in tax to the Mujahideen forces.

Under the protection of the CIA and the Pakistani Inter-Services Intelligence agency (ISI), the Pakistani military and Afghan resistance opened heroin labs on the border of the North West Frontier of Pakistan and Afghanistan. At the end of the Cold War the United States and the USSR both announced the termination of aid to Afghanistan. Afghan guerrillas began a rapid expansion of poppy growing and heroin production.

After the final Soviet withdrawl in 1989, the resulting power vacuum caused rival warlords and factions to fight against each other for power, resulting to ever more opium production to fund their military equipment and activities.

During Taliban rule of Afghanistan from 1996 to 2001, opium output peaked at 4,500 tons in 1999, but in 2000 Taliban leader Mullah Mohammed Omar collaborated with the UN to eradicate heroin production, declaring that growing poppies was un-Islamic. The Taliban then enforced a ban on poppy farming with force and public punishment.

The result was a 99% reduction of poppy farming in Taliban controlled areas. This also resulted in economic devastation for the country, contributing to its status as the sixth poorest country in the world. This in turn arguably made it easier for western military forces to persuade the population to rebel against the regime.

The Taliban was deposed in 2002 as part of a coalition of over 40 countries, including all NATO members, in order to deny al-Qaeda a safe base of operations in Afghanistan after the attacks of the 11th September 2001.

The US had attempted to impose a crop eradication programme in 2004, but the US ambassador to Afghanistan, Zalmay Khalizad, and Ashraf Ghani (who would later become president) warned that widespread impoverishment would further destabilise the region.

Governor Ustad Atta Mohammad Noor achieved a complete eradication in the Balkh Province of Afghanistan from 18,000 hectares (44,478 acres) in 2005 to zero in 2007.

At the peak of its opium production in 2007, the Golden Crescent region produced more than 8,000 of the world's 9,000 tons of opium. Efforts to capture, seize, and intercept opium products have been been unsuccessful, with only around 1% of total production being seized and destroyed, due to bribery and corruption of officials, and many drug traffickers allegedly becoming top officials in the Afghan government of Hamid Karzai.

The destruction of a major drug production site near Jalalabad in October of 2010 by Russian, Afghan, and US anti-drug forces, along with heroin and opium with a street value of $250 million, was a sign of increased cooperation between nations to stamp out the trade. However, this was criticised by Hamid Karzai as a violation of Afghan sovereignty and international law.

8.13 Today

The second largest producer of opium, by size of poppy fields, is Myanmar (Burma) with around 33,100 hectares (81,791 acres) followed by Mexico with around 28,000 hectares (69,189 acres). Poppy fields in other countries add up to around 44,475 hectares (109,900 acres).

But by far the largest producer of opium in the world is Afghanistan with around 224,000 hectares (553,516 acres), rapidly increasing by as much as 37% in a single year according to the Afghanistan Opium Survey carried out by coalition forces and the UN.

Two thirds of the provinces in Afghanistan are directly affected by poppy cultivation, which requires more manpower than other crops, employing more people in the process, in a country where unemployment is at around 40%.

For many, poppy cultivation is seen as the quickest and most effective way to feed their families and keep away the very real threat of poverty, in a country with such harsh and unforgiving mountainous terrain, stretched supply lines, and isolated communities.

Between 80% and 90% of the world's illicit supply of opium originates from Afghanistan, an estimated 6,300 tonnes, making up around 20% of Afghanistan's GDP. Most of the opium from Afghanistan makes its way to Europe via Turkey and the Balkans. 90% of the illicit supply to the UK arrives in this way.

The US is estimated to have spent more than $8.6 billion (£6.3 billion) attempting to halt the opium trade, and continued attempts to educate farmers to grow alternative crops have previously seen limited success. There has been some hope, however, in the form of saffron, a spice which is more expensive than gold. Its cultivation has increased making Afghanistan the third largest saffron producer in the world behind Iran and India.

On the 15th August 2021, Taliban forces captured Kabul, the capital city of Afghanistan. This was the result of an offensive that began in May 2021 against the Afghan government, following the NATO withdrawal of troops from Afghanistan which began on 29th February 2021 with a provisional deadline of the 31st August 2021.

The Taliban stated that there will be "no drug production, no drug smuggling", but that they "need international help for that", implying that they are willing to collaborate with the international community in order to make that happen.

Most countries are not willing to acknowledge the Taliban as the legitimate rulers of Afghanistan, and are heavily sceptical about whether or not they genuinely intend to eliminate opium production, since it has been such a significant income for the Taliban, and a vital economic support for the population they seek to rule over.

In weighing up the pros and cons of the opium trade in the region, perhaps the strongest internal case against the economic argument is that the number of drug users in Afghanistan is estimated to be as high as 2.5 million, including the child labourers who harvest the poppies, combined with the notion that drug use and its intoxication is un-Islamic as declared by religious-political figures.

As long as there is conflict, necessitating rivals to arm themselves against each other, relying on the most effective funding source available, and as long as corruption undermines consistent and fair enforcement, motivating officials to offer protection in return for profit from the illicit economy progress is unlikely.

8.14 Popular Culture

1939   In the film The Wizard of Oz, the Wicked Witch of the West conjures up a poppy field in front of the Emerald City to make Dorothy, the Lion, the Tin Man and the Scarecrow fall asleep, preventing them from entering

1948   Laudanum is portrayed as the surgical drug of choice for fifteenth-century physicians in Lawrence Schoonover's novel The Burnished Blade, the plot of which deals in part with the smuggling of expensive raw opium into France from the Empire of Trebizond.

1960   Harper Lee - To Kill a Mockingbird, features a Caucasian middle-class heroine who becomes addicted to opium after it is prescribed for medicinal use.

1975   Laudanum is prescribed in Glendon Swarthout's novel The Shootist to the character J.B. Books, played by John Wayne in Don Siegel's movie adaptation of 1976

1984   In the film Once Upon a Time in America, the character David 'Noodles' Aaronson (Robert De Niro) frequents an opium den.

1994   In the film Interview with the Vampire, based on the 1976 novel, Claudia uses laudanum to try and dispose of Lestat: Under the pretext of making peace, she offers him some drunk noble-blood twins to feed on, when she has actually had them overdosed with laudanum.

2001   In the film adaptation of From Hell, the main character, Inspector Fred Abberline played by Johnny Depp, frequents opium dens, and uses absinthe laced with laudanum.

2001   In the film Apocalypse Now Redux, a scene that was not included in the original 1979 release shows Captain Benjamin Willard (Martin Sheen) and Roxanne Sarrault (Aurore Clément) smoking an opium pipe.

2002   The film Gangs of New York portrayed rival political ward bosses in search of fraudulent voters rousting Chinese immigrants from an opium den in the Five Points neighborhood of Manhattan, in the 1860s.

2010   In Boardwalk Empire episode 'Nights in Ballygran', Jimmy Darmody is shown smoking opium at an opium den in Chinatown.

2011   Starz Channel Original Series The Borgias. Juan visits an opium den for pain in his leg from a mysterious disease picked up while in the 'new world'.

2013   The TV series 'Peaky Blinders' shows the main character Tommy Shelby using an opium pipe in the very first episode to try and help him sleep without flashbacks of fighting in the trenches of World War I

Sources and Further Reading

Books

Beeching, J.	(1975)	*The Chinese Opium Wars*	1st ed	Harvest	0-15-617094-9
Halpern, J. H. MD, Blistein, D	(2020)	*Opium: How an Ancient Flower Shaped and Poisoned our World*	1st ed	Hachette	978-0-316-41767-9
Inglis, B.	(2017)	*The Opium War*	2017 ed	Endeavour Ink	978-1-911445-92-0
Inglis, L.	(2018)	*Milk of Paradise: A History of Opium*	9th ed	Picador	978-1-4472-8611-0
Lee, P.	(2006)	*Opium Culture: The Art & Ritual of the Chinese Tradition*	10th ed	Park Street	978-1-59477-075-3
Lovell, J.	(2011)	*The Opium War*	2012 ed	Picador	978-0-330-45748-4
Martin, S.	(2012)	*Opium Fiend: A 21st Century Slave to a 19th Century Addiction*	1st ed	Villard	9780345517852
McCoy, A. W.	(1973)	*The Politics of Heroin in Southeast Asia*	80th ed	Harper & Row	06-090328-7
Wigal, D.	(2014)	*Opium: The Flowers of Evil*	1st ed	Parkstone	978-1-78310-018-7

Articles

Sinclair, A. [Forthcoming, late 2021]. High Times in Ancient Egypt: The Use and Abuse of Psychoactive Plant Identifications in Alternative / Pseudo-Egyptology.

Online Articles

Salavert, A., Zazzo, A., Martin, L. et al. Direct dating reveals the early history of opium poppy in western Europe. Sci Rep 10, 20263 (2020). https://doi.org/10.1038/s41598-020-76924-3

Sinclair, A. [Updated April 2021]. *Hul Gil and the opium poppy: A comedy of errors* [online]. Available from: http://artisticlicenseorwhyitrustnoone.blogspot.com/2020/12/hul-gil-and-opium-poppy-comedy-of-errors.html [Accessed July 2021].